SEX ADDICTION CURE

HOW TO OVERCOME PORN ADDICTION AND SEXUAL COMPULSION

MATT PEPLIŃSKI

PsychoTao

Tczew, Malczewskiego 2 83-110, Poland

PsychoTao
Malczewskiego 2
Tczew, Poland/83-110
Psychotao.com

Ordering Information:
Quantity sales. Special discounts are available on quantity purchases by corporations, associations, and others. For details, contact the "Special Sales Department" at empiricspirit@gmail.com

Sex Addiction Cure/ Matt Pepliński. —1st ed.
ISBN 978-83-939027-0-5

CONTENTS

I know this book has a lot of meditations and going through them all can be overwhelming at first. That's why giving you a 90% discount on my home study course to help you build some momentum towards your recovery. You can claim by going to:

Listen, I'm no social scientist and haven't done a survey. I don't pretend to know what John Q citizen thinks about this. But I've lived in prison for a long time now and I've met a lot of men who were motived to commit violence just like me. And without expectation, every one of them was deeply involved in pornography. Without question, without expectation. Deeply influenced and consumed by an addiction to pornography.
-Ted Bundy during an interview with James Dobson (1989) hours before his execution.

[1]

The True Face of Porn.

IN ORDER to effectively cope with any addiction, you first have to understand it. People tend to underestimate the power an addiction has over them, (Alquist and Baumeister, 2012) and this is one of the major reasons why interventions are unsuccessful. (Margolis and Zweben, 2011). A study conducted on smokers (Alquist and Baumeister, 2012, Margolis and Zweben, 2011) has found that people who were the most successful with quitting smoking not only understood how smoking negatively affected their life, but they also understood the mechanism of how their addiction took power over them. This allowed them to understand that quitting an addiction requires a lot of understanding as well as effort. Not taking the time to do both will slow down the recovery process if not halt it completely

EVOLUTION HAS NOT PREPARED US FOR PORN.

Pornography overloads the dopamine receptors in our brain, which leads to numerous after effects. This is also why it's so addicting. Internet porn is particularly problematic. In the past, porn addiction was not as much of a problem, because when you bought a Playboy or a Penthouse, you didn't really see the kind of hardcore stuff you have on the internet. If you were really obsessed with porn and had the extra money, you could maybe watch 10 women per hour. On the internet with a fast connection, you can easily watch over hundreds of pictures per hour. In an experiment, rats were given numerous sexual partners. They have found out that rats could have sex indefinitely if they always had it with a different sexual partner. This effect has been called the **Coolidge Effect** and Porn emulates it. When you browse over hundreds of naked bodies in succession while masturbating, your brain thinks you're having sex with the figures in front of your monitor, and due to the Coolidge effect you can do this for hours and hours. This produces very negative brain changes that were never seen prior to the Internet.

LET'S DISCUSS HOW PORN TURNS YOUR BRAIN INTO AN ADDICTED BRAIN

All addictions create pathological changes in your brain's structure. Porn addiction for example directly lowers activity in the orbitofrontal cortex, which is responsible for making strategic decisions, rather than impulsive ones. (Watts and Hilton, 2011) A 2007 study on porn addiction demonstrated measurable volume loss in several areas of the brain mostly in the frontal lobes (the area of the brain responsible for impulse control). In short, the study found that porn addiction can cause physical, anatomical change in the brain, the hallmark of brain addiction. (Watts and Hilton, 2011)

In 2005. Dr. Eric Nestler proposed the theory that all addictions occur when the pleasure/reward pathways in the brain are hijacked. Porn use, like other abusable substances, modifies them directly. For example, DeltaFosB is a protein that's over-expressed in the brains of addicts. It's over expression is also found in porn addicts. It's now a fact that porn addiction creates real negative changes in your brain. (Watts and Hilton, 2011)

It is now clinically understood that dopamine is the common denominator in all addictions. With any addiction, your dopamine pathways become desensitized. For example, cocaine and heroin are addicting because they artificially increase levels of dopamine. By masturbating for hours, your brain is flooded with dopamine.

Dopamine is responsible for motivation, and once you become desensitized to it you need more of it to get the same effect. This is why after prolonged porn-use, your brain needs not only more porn to get aroused but also has a harder time to get motivated by anything else.

While porn in one form or another has been available for 200 years, never before in human history were we able to watch thousands of women in succession in 100 tabs in a browser for free. When we do that, our brains become flooded with dopamine, which overloads our dopamine receptors, which in turn makes us demotivated, prone to depression, and causes numerous sexual problems.

6 CORE COMPONENTS OF ADDICTION

Some people doubt that porn addiction is a legitimate addiction. Let's now discuss the components of addiction and see if porn addiction fits in them. (Clarkson and Kopaczewski, 2013)

1. Your thoughts become dominated by - The object of your addiction. If you cannot stop thinking about porn. That's a basic sign for addiction.

2. Your mood changes when - You succumb to your addiction. If you're angry at yourself after you relapse or if you feel guilty.

3. Tolerance - You need more of it in order to get the same high. If you progressed from vanilla pornography to more hardcore pornography to get the same effects as before that's another sign to watch out for.

4. **Withdrawal Symptoms - You feel bad when you quit for a while and you feel like "need" more in order to continue normally with your daily life.**
5. **Conflict - Your addiction negatively influences your life and those around you, and you want to stop but can't, no matter how much you try or how hard people insist you quit.**
6. **Relapse - If you can't stop yourself from using pornography, and you relapse to it even if you don't want to.**

As you can see, just about any addiction can be easily interchangeable with all of these. Porn addiction is a reality and it should be treated the same way any other common addiction.

Let's Discuss How Porn Addiction Influences Development

Neglect during childhood predisposes you to addiction because the parts of the brain responsible for impulse control become underdeveloped. (Watts and Hilton, 2011)

Neglected children produce less dopamine since they can't naturally meet their brains needs for dopamine, they often look to outside sources to get this need met. For many trauma victims, addiction becomes a survival strategy. During trauma, the amygdala becomes hypersensitive. Porn becomes a way to self-medicate. (Watts and Hilton, 2011)

Shame has been found to be linked to porn and sex addiction. The more you resist an emotion, the stronger it gets. Someone ashamed of his sexual behavior unknowingly strengthens its grip over him.

PORN WRECKS YOUR SEXUALITY

Porn is like drugs in many ways. Many people start with marijuana and then progress to crack and other harsher drugs because they need a better 'high'. Porn overloads your dopamine receptors in a similar way and many porn addicts search for a stronger 'high' to get off to. That's why so many porn addicts develop fetishes. I myself developed quite a number of fetishes because I watched porn during the crucial years of my development. This applies to both men and women. My first serious long distance girlfriend was a very avid porn user. She started at an early age too, and also with soft-core porn at first, then she progressed to porn involving urination, and then to zoophilia. And in her case, this progressed to real life deviancies, like masturbating dogs on the street. Fetishes often become harder to manage because our brain identifies nonsexual images as porn and those images aren't seen as porn by most people. In my case, even a lot of nonsexual pictures on art websites were pornographic for me and not filtered through the site's mature filter. That's why I had to use a porn blocker in a very specific way to block those images. Luckily porn induced fetishes eventually go away when you stop watching porn for about 2 years or so.

NOW LET ME TELL YOU HOW PORN RUINED MY LIFE.

Now that I've introduced you to my ex-girlfriend, lets discuss a bit more about my personal life. Keep in mind the details ahead of you are explicit in nature, but as someone that survived through pornography addiction, I need to let you know these gross details so you'll have an idea how drastic it can be, and I am not the worse example when it comes to this. I know very well how destructive porn can be, I know that due to the current state of our culture, there will be always a nagging voice that will tell you 'oh porn is not so bad', 'porn is cool', 'there's nothing wrong with porn'. For most of my life, I used to think this way.

I was a shut in all my life. I mean, I learned English because I did nothing else as a kid but watch cartoons on cartoon network (which was in English in Poland).

When I was a teenager, I had pretty severe anxiety issues so I didn't leave my house and didn't have many friends. In a way, porn was my only friend, and as such I often went out of my way to search for porn and collected it. At one point, I had 1TB of pornographic comics and videos. I even was a fairly active part of a pornographic subculture called the "furry community". By being part of the pornographic side from that culture, I even began to self-identify as a "furry".

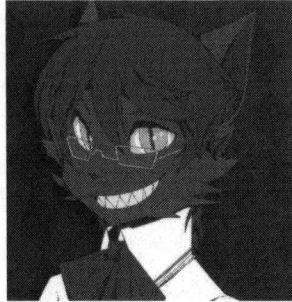

As shown here, my former "fursona".

My entire social network was composed of porn users and porn artists. All of my friends on my friend list not only prolifically used porn, but were avid fans of it, like a religious movement. In fact, my aforementioned girlfriend was a porn artist that was quite famous in the furry community.

So as you can see, at one point in my life I really didn't see anything bad in porn. In fact, I thought it was the greatest thing on the planet. But things changed when I actually wanted to get real sexual intimacy. It was only then that the problems around pornography became clear.

First and foremost, I developed something called Post Orgasmic Illness Syndrome.

Post orgasmic illness syndrome (POIS) can be defined essentially as feeling sick after ejaculation/orgasm, much like a hangover. Since I was 16, I began to feel sick for a week each time I ejaculated. For me, it was a profound sickness. Imagine having flu and multiply it 10 times. It was quite debilitating and it stopped me from functioning at school, causing me to fail high school. Not even this stopped me from using porn; in fact it just propelled my addiction.

"What else do I have?" I said to myself. Even after I somehow managed to get to university, I still used porn. I masturbated and masturbated, obsessing over my fantasies. Feeling sick after using pornography didn't stop me at all. As I've mentioned before, it was just like a bad hangover, it was very problematic, but when you're an alcoholic you really struggle to stop after a while, you even lose touch of what matters to you most.

Porn is a drug, it's not only addicting but you actually need a stronger "fix" each time you use it. When I first started using porn, I was disgusted by anything but the most soft-core porn. But after only a few years of using porn, I developed numerous disturbing fetishes. Being a furry was the least freaky thing I was into. Here's a short list of things I once masturbated to on a regular basis:

WEIGHT GAIN PORN – its porn in which a woman deliberately fattens herself to obesity. I would spend hours on the internet searching for stories and comics about the subject so I would satisfy my needs. Oddly enough, whenever I found a girl who was "into that sort of thing" on a dating site, I would never initiate contact. I would just masturbate to her profile picture. I'm noting this because I want you to know that having a similar fetish is not something that will really "get you dates". These kinds of people don't care about any of that. The ones that do are not generally looking for long-term intimate relationships with people that share their fetishes online, like my first girlfriend for instance.

AMPUTEE PORN – I began to experience full sexual gratification only when I saw a woman suffer and powerless. I began to look for and masturbate to comics depicting women without arms and legs.

OMORASHI/URINATION – This was actually directly related to the one "relationship" I got out of my porn addiction. Once while scouring a furry dating website, I've met a girl that would become my first girlfriend. She was the only person I've met that was more into porn than I was. She was actually obsessed with it. In fact, she was on disability and lived with her parents because she did nothing else but draw and masturbate. She flunked out of community college and essentially spent her days masturbating to urination porn online. She was admittedly a long distance relationship and our relationship was very much centered on pornography. Ultimately, she didn't really like me for what I was, she just wanted to satisfy her sexual needs, and I obliged. I urinated myself for her repeatedly just to cater to her fetishes. Eventually she became bored with me and abandoned me. Today, I know that this is the best kind of "relationship" (Love and friendship wise) you'll get if you try to find people through porn instead of developing intimacy: A cheap meaningless fling at best.

After that experience, I became serious about quitting porn. That was no easy feat. I actually noticed that I couldn't get an erection without pornography, which is something many long-term porn users experience. Of course my POIS was still present, and due to extensive porn use, I conditioned in myself a very strong case of premature ejaculation. psychotherapy.

I've tried everything to recover:

Psychotherapy

Psychiatrists

Counselors

Forums

But nothing really helped. Only after years of trial and error, which involved me getting a BSC in psychology, I was able to help myself with my porn addiction. In this book I'll save you years (and a fortune in student loans) by putting everything that I found helpful into a step-by-step system that's guaranteed to help you overcome your porn addiction if you follow the steps I'll provide you with.

WHY IS PORN ADDICTING?

Addicting things are addicting because they trigger a dopamine release by mimicking natural responses to things like sex and food. Porn plays around with your dopamine receptors just like any addictive drug. (Watts and Hilton, 2011) Most porn addicts start watching porn at a very early age because porn equals instant gratification. It's a quick and easy escape. Most addictions are all about escaping something: grief, low self-esteem, anger, hatred. I used porn to escape from depression and low self-esteem as well as self-medication.

Addictions in general also makes you more predisposed to develop other addictions. This is why porn users are often also addicted to other things, like video games and drugs for example.

HOW PORN MAKES YOU DEPRESSED

Dopamine is the neurotransmitter that determines how motivated we are to do things. Repeated porn use messes up our dopamine, so it also messes up our motivation. (Watts and Hilton, 2011)

Not all instances of depression are caused or linked with porn, but all instances of depression are relieved when you stop using porn. Luckily, when you stop using porn your dopamine receptors recover their sensitivity. It will take months, but the changes will be noticeable in the very first month. The problematic thing though is that the depression caused by porn makes it harder for you to resist the urge to watch porn. It impairs the communication between your prefrontal cortex and the hippocampus, making the addiction very hard to beat on your own. (Watts and Hilton, 2011)

HOW PORN MAKES YOU STUPID

Concentration is the ability to choose what you want to focus on and ignore stuff that's irrelevant.

Extensive porn use destroys your ability to concentrate because it forces your brain to categorize normal things as unimportant. When your dopamine receptors become desensitized, they need a greater stimulation to become aroused, and as such you find it hard to concentrate on 'normal' things such as reading for example.

This desensitization also messes up your hippocampus. The hippocampus plays a very important part in the formation of long term memories. As such extensive porn use also messes up your memory. (Watts and Hilton, 2011)

I know from brain scans that my hippocampus is very small due to my extensive porn use and a life long struggle with depression (which I've won by the way). But my shrunken hippocampus didn't make my life into a real live version of Memento though. It just made it harder for me to prepare for my exams, remember people's names, etc.

HOW PORN DESTROYS RELATIONSHIPS

Your brain learns terrible lessons about relationships and sex from porn. For example, porn causes intrusive sexual thoughts, which can lead to fetishes, paraphilias, depression, erectile dysfunction, loss of concentration, and lower self-esteem, making it harder to attract women. Women are very often disgusted by what porn promotes and know when you are looking at them the same way you view porn actresses, and are repelled and even repulsed by it. Porn-caused erectile dysfunction doesn't help either and many porn users find that they can't get it up in bed. The good thing is that once you quit porn for an extended period your sex will change from mere fornication into love making. From lust to intimacy. When you do porn, you condition your brain to be aroused to porn alone. Some porn users actually start 'preferring' porn to real life sex.

I can give you a personal story of mine. When I was in the furry community, I once had a friend that claimed to be asexual, but really this person was just a porn addict who couldn't get it up unless he masturbated to pornography. He did masturbate to porn for several hours a day, even though he was 'asexual'. Extensive porn use has been found to directly cause erectile dysfunction. This is why erectile dysfunction is now more common among 20 year olds than ever before. (McDougal and Hannesson, n.d.). When you're sexually aroused, your brain creates a chemical called cGMP which causes erections. When you're desensitized to dopamine due to extensive porn use, very little cGMP is produced and you can't get it up. Neither Viagra nor other erectile pills will help. (Watts and Hilton, 2011) To test whether or not porn caused your erectile dysfunction simply try and masturbate without any porn or sexual fantasy. If you can't get erect to physical self-stimulation, but can get erect to porn, then you've got a porn-induced erectile dysfunction. But thankfully all of this is completely reversible if you quit porn for an extended amount of time.

PORN ALSO NEGATIVELY IMPACTS DATING

Here's a quick checklist to further determine if you're addicted to porn:

- Have you taken a day off work or opted out of social events so you could stay home and watch porn?
- When you finish watching porn, are you ashamed?
- Have you lied to your spouse or family about how much porn you watch, or about what kinds of porn you watch?
- Have you unsuccessfully tried to reduce or stop your porn use?
- Do you have problems focusing or anything that isn't sexualized?
- Have you accessed porn from work, school or a public place?
- Did porn cause you problems at work?
- Do you get frustrated when you want to use porn but can't?
- Do you spend more time on porn than you would like?
- Do you have problems getting out of bed without using porn first?
- Has a spouse or family member complained about the amount of time you spend online?

If you answered yes to any of these questions. You're a porn addict.

WHAT CONTRIBUTES TO PORN ADDICTION?

Study after study has found that people whom suffer from isolation are more suggestible to addictions of any kind, and porn addicts tend to be isolated. (Owens, Behun, Manning and Reid, 2012, Rosenberg and Kraus, 2014)

Stress is also a major contributor. In fact for most people, stress seems to be their main trigger. (Owens, Behun, Manning and Reid, 2012, Rosenberg and Kraus, 2014)

Remember: One addiction predisposes you to others. If you're addicted to an addiction then you're more likely to become addicted to porn and vice versa (Watts and Hilton, 2011)

YOU DON'T HAVE TO LIKE DOING PORN

The brain systems that are responsible for 'liking' and 'wanting' are separate systems. An addiction influences the 'wanting' mechanisms.(Watts and Hilton, 2011) That's how one can actually be addicted to masturbating to a fetish one doesn't even like. For example I was addicted to weight gain porn, even though I didn't even like it. I in fact hated it and that didn't make much of a difference.

WHAT MAKES PORN SO DANGEROUS

- Firstly sex and porn cause people to ignore obvious dangers. For example; Think of the pedophiles and pederast that risks everything to satisfy their needs or the people that spends hundreds and even thousands in dollars to get their pornographic fix.
- Additionally porn is everywhere. Unlike an alcoholic or drug addict, you have a steady and free supply to your drug.
- Society promotes porn. Popular media is very sexualized.
- Porn can escalate into paraphilias. Having an antisocial paraphilia is not functional.
- You carry your own source of supply in your smart phone or laptop.

You Might Experience Withdrawal Symptoms

Porn addiction like every addiction has withdrawal symptoms. Example withdrawal symptoms include:

- Irritability
- Jitters
- Itchy skin
- Genital discomfort
- Restlessness
- Headaches
- Anxiety

Different people experience different withdrawal symptoms. Some experience none, others can experience these and more. We'll help you manage them in this book.

Exercise

I would like you to take a pen and paper and ask yourself these questions:

- How did porn influence your life?
- How did porn influence your emotions and social life?
- How much time have you wasted on porn?

[2]

Porn Blocking That Works

MOST FREE PORN BLOCKING techniques don't work because if you're addicted to porn and install a free porn blocker like K9 Web Protection, it won't take you long to find some way to bypass it. In a typical situation, you'll be the one installing the blocker, and so you'll know your own password. You'll be able to turn it off with a single click. So what's the solution?

BLOCKING INTERNET ACCESS THROUGH COLD TURKEY

Cold turkey is a productivity app that most people use to block websites like Facebook for a week. However, this is not how you will use it in this book. You'll use it to block off internet completely for a period time daily along with completely blocking your most dangerous websites You can get it at: getcoldturkey.com

The idea is that you don't really need to use your computer 24/7, and you can always completely block access to your most risky websites. With the pro version of cold turkey, you'll be able to block your access to your browser during certain hours: The hours which you're the most prone to relapse (we'll help you identify them in a future lesson). It will also allow you to set up another group of websites which you can block for a specific amount of time..

BLOCKING INTERNET ACCESS USING K9

K9 Web Protection (www.k9webprotection.com) is free software that will also allow us to block internet access for you during specific times of day. Let me again explain the rationale behind this:

We each have times when we're most relapse prone, I for example am most suggestible to relapse before 2pm and after 9pm. This is when my stress levels are the highest. If you don't know your 'relapse times', don't worry. Further in this book, you'll be asked to keep a journal to help you determine exactly when you're most prone to use porn.

It's also important to note that most of the time porn addiction is not only porn addiction, it's also internet addiction. Studies have shown that nothing makes you less productive than the internet; as such the simplest and most powerful way to improve your productivity and set yourself up for success is to simply limit your internet access to periods where you actually need to use the internet. It's that simple. With that simple technique you'll easily eliminate 50% of internet porn from your life.

Multiple studies have shown that the Internet is the biggest time and productivity drain on the planet. Do you really need it on 24/7? That's why I want you to block your Internet access for most of the day. If you already know roughly when you're most prone to using porn, I would suggest you block internet access during those times.

I want you to try this and you'll be amazed how much your productivity will increase once you get rid of the greatest distraction known on planet earth – the Internet.

This is not to say that you won't be able to use the internet for productive means. You will. I currently work completely online, and I'm able to do this with only a 4 hour internet window. In fact, I wrote this book while being able to access the internet only for 4 hours per day. I simply schedule the work I have to do online during that time period, and do it then. This also makes sure I don't have time online to spend on porn.

EXERCISE

- During what time period(s) are you most prone to relapse on porn?
- Would it be possible for you to be internet free during those times?
- What productive things would you do during your internet/porn free time?

It's been proven that we're the most productive when we're free from distractions. I would like you to pick at least a few high-priority tasks that you can do offline during your 'internet free' period. If you're a programmer, you could be typing out the code for a project offline, and if you're a web designer you could test and code your website on a local server installation.

[3]

The Scientific Basis of This Book

I WANT TO DEVOTE, this lesson to explaining the science behind this book.

This book is based on ACT which stands for Acceptance and Commitment Therapy:

There have been numerous studies which have shown ACT (which itself is an evolution of Cognitive Behavioral Therapy) (González-Menéndez, Fernández, Rodríguez, & Villagrá, 2014) to be an effective treatment for all forms of addiction. (Kelly et al., 2015)

I want note that every serious therapy will require a great deal of effort on your part. This is the only way we'll be able to properly redirect your habits for the better.

This might seem like a lot to you, because most self-help programs don't require you to do much of anything. But this is because most other self-help programs don't treat change seriously. Most self-help programs are not personally accountable for your change. They just give you some motivation, some affirmation and some common sense 'life lessons'. Because they generally deal with minor problems like "oh I feel a little down". But here, our priority is for you to change your behavior for the better. This is a serious program that's designed for serious change.

Additionally, many self-help programs try to make you 'feel better' or 'take all of your urges away' instantaneously. This is not realistic. In the beginning, you will feel urges to do porn. They will subside in time, but in the beginning they'll be there.

That's why the goal of the NoPorn Plan, ACT (on which the NoPorn Plan is based upon) and evidence-based psychotherapy in general is not to make you feel better. It's to make you ACT even when you feel like terrible, and even when you feel the strong urge to do porn. This is what psychologists call Psychological Flexibility. (Webb, Beard, Kertz, Hsu, & Björgvinsson, 2016) This term just means that you'll able to take action in a way you'll enjoy no matter how you feel or what happens inside of your mind.

Let's elaborate some more on the definition of psychological flexibility. Psychological flexibility is the ability to do whatever you choose to do, whenever you choose to do it, without being limited in your choices by what's inside of your head. Like giving a speech to a large group of people, you might feel anxiety and a negative internal dialogue, but with psychological flexibility you'd be able to do it no matter what.

It's all about not letting yourself be controlled by the thoughts in your head and all about pro-actively deciding what you want to do. It's not about trying to control these urges or thoughts. It's about being able to experience them and still act in a way that's in alignment with your values. For you as a porn addict it means being able to feel the urge to do porn and do productive stuff instead.

That's why guided self-development exercises will be such a crucial part of this program. These exercises will allow you to stop and notice the automatic thoughts that make you do porn, even if you don't want to. When you slow down and remain still, you might notice thoughts like: "It'll just be this one porn comic, and I'll stop. I had a terrible experience today, and I really need this comic to take the edge off. I feel so alone, I don't want to be alone anymore, porn will make me feel as if I have a lover of my own."

Make no mistake: these thoughts are painful, and powerful. It's natural for you to want to run from them, but if you become mindful you'll be able to just recognize these thoughts as thoughts and act consciously in a way that you want to, which is not to succumb to them.

LET'S AGAIN RECAP PSYCHOLOGICAL FLEXIBILITY:

Your mind says you can't do it?

When you practice psychological flexibility you do it anyway.

You feel like you can't do anything.

When you practice psychological flexibility you do what you need to anyway.

Of course this might sound simple. But to 'do it anyway', you need to develop something I call your mindfulness muscle.

Our brains never unlearn things, and as such to be able to take control of your mind you have to learn something new. You need to learn something that will allow you to resist being controlled by negative emotions and thoughts. These skills are what psychologists call mindfulness skills.

I know you've tried to quit porn before. What happened the last time you didn't want to masturbate to porn, but did it anyway? Ask yourself these questions:

- What did your mind tell you?
- What happened in your mind?
- What emotions did you feel in your body?

You might not remember, and you might not have noticed before. That's why in this program you'll learn to slow down. So that you'll be able to catch these thoughts and emotions. Because in order to become free from them, you first have to become aware of them. Usually these thoughts are like "Oh porn isn't so bad. What's wrong with just letting loose a bit? By masturbating to fetish porn you're re-affirming your sexuality."

I want to state the obvious here: These thoughts are SCARY. They are powerful. They can take control of you. It's only natural for you to want to escape from them. But after practicing mindfulness techniques you'll learn in this book for a while, you'll learn to recognize these thoughts as what they are: thoughts that don't have to control you if you don't want them to. In time, you'll be able to choose what you wanted all along, which is not to masturbate to porn among other things.

Most traditional forms of CBT focus on changing your thoughts. We also do this here, but we go beyond that. We give you tools that will allow you to transcend your thoughts, and stop being a slave to them. You will achieve this by training 6 mindfulness skills through a regular practice of mindfulness.

LET'S NOW LOOK AT THESE MINDFULNESS SKILLS ONE BY ONE.

1. **COGNITIVE DEFUSION** – This skill allow you to be aware of a thought/emotion without being controlled by it. In this book you'll learn various mindfulness exercises which will train you to notice your thoughts without acting on them. Slowly this will train you in being able to feel your urges to masturbate to porn, without acting on them. It's not about controlling your thoughts or emotions. It's all about being aware of them and being able to be free from their control and free to respond in a way that's aligned with your values.

2. **WILLINGNESS** - Most people use porn because they want to escape certain other negative emotions. Various mindfulness techniques such emotional labeling or Trauma Releasing Exercises will help you with the skill of embracing life as it is.

3. PRESENT MOMENT AWARENESS - When you're in the present moment, you're at your maximum capacity. Pretty much every mindfulness exercise in this book will gradually train you in this skill.

4. UNDERSTANDING THAT YOU'RE NOT YOUR THOUGHTS - We are attached to our stories, our conceptualized self. We think that WE ARE our porn addiction, WE ARE our stories, WE ARE a diagnostic category. By understanding that you're not your stories and self-judgements, you'll learn how to be free from them and they'll stop fueling your addictions. This skill is mostly trained by the various worksheets you're required to complete during this book and your journal.

5. VALUED LIVING - In order to live a meaningful life, you'll need to know what's meaningful to you. By identifying your values, you'll have something more important and fulfilling to do than masturbating to porn. This will give you the motivation and drive to quit your habit once and for all.

6. COMMITMENT - In this book you'll learn how to set goals according ot your values and carry them out responsibility.

In this book you'll also learn other skills that are specifically required to beat porn addiction. You'll learn how to identify your triggers and manage them through techniques such as **TAAP**, Urge Surfing and others. You'll also learn dating, relationship and sexuality skills. The last part of the NoPorn Plan is designed to give you what porn has taken away: Your ability to naturally attract a worthwhile partner, and be able to have a functional and intimate relationship with them. This is achievable through a technique I call the "Porn Trauma Release", which you'll learn later in the book. In short: MINDFULNESS + VALUES + ACTION = PSYCHOLOGICAL FLEXIBILITY

You will create new get a script for mindfulness through breathing. This exercise has been used to train mindfulness for millennia, and will help you develop mindfulness skills if you'll practice it regularly. If you want a recorded version of this please go to

http://nopornplan.com

You will also get a free video series and comic book that will build upon the things you've learned in this book

MINDFULNESS OF BREATHING

Please find a quiet place free from any distractions. Sit with your spine straight and either close your eyes or have them lightly open, focused on a spot in front of you. Optionally if you have back problems you can lay on a flat surface with your hands on your sides and with your head supported by a pillow.

Allow yourself to turn your attention to your breathing, and observe it as if you're a curious scientist who has never encountered breathing before.

Pause for 5 seconds

Notice the air as it comes in through your nostrils

Pause again for 5 seconds

And notice as it flows back out again

Pause for 5 seconds

Follow it as it goes all the way in and all the way out

Pause for 10 seconds

Notice how the air moves in and out of your nostrils. Notice how it's slightly warmer as it comes out... and slightly cooler as it goes in. Notice the subtle rise and fall of your shoulders...

Pause for 5 seconds

Notice the gentle rise and fall of your rib cage. Just notice it. Rising and falling.

Pause for 5 seconds

Notice the rise and fall of your abdomen. Rising as you breathe in and falling as you breathe out. This shows you that you're breathing from the diaphragm

Pause for 5 seconds

Fix your attention on one of these areas, whichever you prefer: on the breath moving in and out of the nostrils, or on the rising and falling of your abdomen or rib cage

Pause for 5 seconds

Keep your attention on this spot, noticing the movement – in and out- of the breath

Pause for 20 seconds

Whenever feelings, urges or sensations arise, whether pleasant or unpleasant, gently acknowledge them, as if nodding your head at people passing by you on the street

Pause for 5 seconds

Gently acknowledge their presence and let them be

Pause for 5 seconds

Allow them to come and go as they please and just keep your attention on your breath

Pause 20 seconds

Inevitably. Your attention will wander and you'll get caught up in your thoughts. Each time that happens, notice what distracted you, and then bring your attention back to the breath

Pause for 20 seconds

No matter how often you drift off, whether a few times or a thousand- your aim is simply to note what distracted you and to return your attention back to your breath

Pause for 10 seconds

Again and again and again you'll drift off into your thoughts. This is normal and happens to everyone. Our minds naturally distract us from what we're doing. So each time you realize your attention has wandered gently acknowledge it, notice what distracted you, and return your attention to the breath

Pause for 20 seconds

If frustration, boredom, anxiety or sadness arises, simply acknowledge them, and return to the breath

Pause for 20 seconds

No matter how often your attention wanders, gently acknowledge it, note what distracted you, whether it was a thought an emotion or a sensation, and then refocus on your breath.

Pause for 10 seconds

Continue doing it on your own for 5 more minutes. I'll tell you when the meditation will end.

After five minutes

When you are ready, bring yourself back to the room and open your eyes

[4]

What Motivates Your Sex and Porn Addiction

AFTER I'LL GIVE YOU A GOOD grounding in mindfulness exercise, I'll teach you how to use these skills to directly handle your pornographic urges. However, to do that you'll first have to become a bit more aware of them and of things that activate them. The things that activate your pornographic urges are called 'triggers'.

Triggers can be places, objects, certain days, even people. They are specific to an individual.

To adequately cope with your porn addiction, you'll have to learn how to identify them and manage them. Some triggers that are places or things, i.e. bars for alcoholics, can be feasibly avoided and for these triggers its best to do so. Other triggers can be circumstantial and be worked with or changed feasibly, E.g. distancing yourself from friends that enjoy drinking while you are trying to stay sober. However there are triggers that cannot be effectively avoided or resolved like stress with work or loneliness and anxiety, so you'll have to learn how to accept and be present with them.

That's why from this point on, in your journal you'll be asked to identify your triggers. This will be a daily activity that will slowly increase your awareness of what makes you turn to porn in the first place, so that you'll be able to prepare for the more advanced relapse-prevention strategies coming up in this book.

HOW TO GET RID OF FETISHES

I also promised you to teach you a way to get rid of fetishes. Well, fetishes are very commonly conditioned through porn use, and will naturally subside once you quit using porn. But at this point of the book, if you find that you have a fetish that is very uncomfortable and you can't yet stop yourself from using porn, then I suggest that you use softcore porn or porn that is of a different, less disturbing fetish. I did this with weight-gain fetishism.

When I was addicted to weight gain porn I have found that it was very hard for me to resist it, that's why initially when my mindfulness skills were low, instead of watching weight-gain porn I started watching feminization and cross-dressing porn. I have found that type of porn to be less disturbing and I found that I had an easier time resisting flashbacks and urges to masturbate to that kind of porn than to weight gain porn.

But of course, if I have trained my mindfulness skills sufficiently, I would not watch porn at all. It really is not too difficult to do so once you start to regularly implement the power block (with Covenant Eyes, Cold Turkey, or K9), the NoPorn Phrase, and the other techniques that you'll learn in this book. You can practice these techniques even while doing other things. For example you can train mindfulness while eating by just putting your whole attention on that activity.

LET'S NOW DO A FEW EXERCISES THAT WILL HELP YOU IDENTIFY YOUR TRIGGERS:

1. Now. Imagine you're about to use porn. Where are you?
I would like you to imagine now that you're about to use porn, and I want you to answer each of these questions based on what you envision. Refer to your past experiences in trying to answer these questions.

2. What would you use to watch porn? Would you use your computer? (Did you remember to install your porn blocker?) Maybe your smartphone? (You can install a porn blocker on that too by the way).

3. What time of day would it be? (This will give you an idea of when to block Internet access altogether, as we discussed in the power block.)

4. What would you be doing immediately before using porn?

5. What emotions would you commonly experience before viewing pornography?

6. What would usually happen before you used porn?

7. In what ways are you putting yourself at risk of relapsing? Are you for example browsing the Internet needlessly? Are you watching R-rated movies that you know that have something that could trigger you?

8. It might be that you're as part of a subculture that reinforces porn use, such as the furry subculture, fetlife, BDSM, BBW, people going out to strip clubs on a regular basis, or other fetish groups. If so they

act as a trigger for you. They are enablers. Is there any way you could limit your involvement in these subcultures? If so how?

9. Many people use addictions to cope with stress, negative emotions and stressful situations. When you think about your future, how could difficult feelings or situations make you relapse on porn? What difficult feelings or situations would it be?

10. Porn also becomes a part of our daily routine. I for example used to always masturbate at 6 pm and not stop until I went to sleep. In your daily routine when are you most vulnerable to relapse? Would it be possible for you to block your internet access at that time?

11. How might you be taking such unnecessary risks? Do you maybe still frequent a raunchy forum? Do you still have a porn stash for an "emergency"? Contemplate this for a while and write it in your answer

Many porn addicts feel the need to 'test' their recovery by putting themselves in situations that used to trigger them. This almost always leads to a relapse. For example, when I was almost recovered from porn I set up an account on deviantart, a major trigger for me. I told myself that I was ' recovered enough' to browse the art on that website without being affected by the fat fetish material found on that site. I was wrong. I was able to use mindfulness and other skills to resist it a few times but after a while of taking such unnecessary risks, I relapsed.

12. Many relapses are triggered by stress. I want you to name a few stressful situations and negative emotions that might trigger a relapse. You'll learn how to better manage and handle your emotions

and urges in future lessons. So stay tuned. Right now we're just becoming more aware.

13. When you experience urges or cravings to act out addictively, how does your body feel?

14. What feelings will place you at the greatest risk for relapse?

Here are some emotions many people escape from through the use of pornography:

- **Anger**
- **Anxiety**
- **Boredom**
- **Sadness**
- **Fatigue**
- **Fear**
- **Loneliness**
- **Self-pity**
- **Shame**

In psychology trying to escape these emotions through porn or other means is called Experiential Avoidance. Often times we simply can't avoid feeling these emotions that's why in future lessons we'll teach you an alternative strategy that has been found to be far more beneficial and effective.

15. This checklist helps you identify factors that strengthen your porn addiction. The higher your score, the more your environment strengthens your porn addictions.

- I hide my porn from others
- I lie to maintain my contact with porn
- I daydream about times when I can use porn
- I am entitled to use as much porn as I want
- I have an addictive nature
- I am related to someone who has a porn problem
- I maintain a stash of pornography
- I turn to porn when I am bored
- I would like to experience the sex I see in porn
- My friends and contacts are also into pornography
- My greatest sexual satisfaction occurs when I am using porn
- I use porn when I am feeling distressed and want to feel better
- I turn to porn instead of real people for comfort
- I continue using porn even though it is inconsistent with my values and beliefs
- I need to use porn or think about it in order to become sexually aroused
- I use porn as my model for how to have sex
- I think about porn images during sex with a real-life partner
- I like porn that features illegal or abusive sexual activities
- I arrange my life to make sure I have regular time to be with porn
- I make sure I always have access to porn whenever I might want it
- I am most attracted to people who look like porn stars
- I need porn as a sexual outlet if I am not in a relationship
- I am uncomfortable with masturbation unless I am using porn or thinking about it
- I prefer using porn alone rather than with a partner
- My sexual interests have become more extreme since using porn
- The possibility I could get caught makes porn use more exciting

16. Lastly, try to come up with 3 triggers or cues that might tell you that you're close to using porn, including ones not on the list.

[5]

To Become Free from Your Sex and Porn Addiction You Need to Make Friends With Uncertainty.

EMOTIONS AND URGES can best be described as quicksand. You might remember an old movie in which a character fell into a pool of quicksand: The more the character struggled the more it sucked him under. In quicksand, the worst thing you can do is to struggle. The best way to survive is to lie back, spread out your arms and legs, and float on the surface. This is very difficult to do because our instincts tell us to struggle, but if you do what comes naturally, you'll drown. You can notice that our emotions work in a similar way. The more you try to resist an emotion or thought, the stronger they get, but at the same time lying back and floating in your emotional and thinking landscape is hard because it's so counterintuitive.

I want to now further elaborate how this issue of control specifically relates to porn addiction:

YOU CAN NEVER FULLY KNOW THAT YOU'LL NEVER RELAPSE

Quitting porn, like any addiction will always carry with itself a very real uncertainty. In the moment when you smash your fist and say, "Never again", vowing that you'll never masturbate to porn again, you'll always feel an uncomfortable feeling of uncertainty within yourself.(Wilson & DuFrene, 2012)

There are many ways in which people try to manage this feeling of uncertainty. Some just try to repeatedly reaffirm that they will "**NEVER DO PORN AGAIN**" and this alone works to an extent. It re-motivates you and reminds you of your commitment. That's why we've incorporated a modified form of affirmation like this in the **TAAP** protocol, which you'll learn in a future lesson. But the problem with affirmations is that they never get rid of this nagging feeling of uncertainty.

Additionally, affirmations and declarations like this are simply over-used and are ultimately not that effective on their own. I can't tell you how many times I've masturbated to the most disgusting fetish porn ever created just to tell myself "I can't believe I did that. I will never masturbate to porn again". Well... actually I can tell you, it's definitively more than a hundred, and it never stopped me from going back to porn.

If this doesn't work, then why is it so common? The reason for this is that when we do it, we sincerely do want to quit porn, another reason is that we say such things primarily to suppress our fears of another relapse. It's yet another attempt to control our thoughts and emotions, which never works. There's even a saying for it "What resists, persists." I'll explain why in this lesson.

There's only one way to truly get rid of this uncertainty, one way to truly answer the question: "Will I ever use porn again?" and that's using porn again. When you use porn again, the uncertainty is removed. You know that you'll masturbate to porn again.

WHENEVER I TRIED TO QUIT PORN I ALWAYS PROMISED MYSELF:

"I'm fed up with this. This is the last time. I'll never masturbate to disgusting weight gain porn again". But there was always a little seed of doubt present. My mind always reminded me:

"But that's what happened last time. You've promised this to yourself numerous times. If it didn't work then, what makes you think it will work now?" And then surely something triggered me, and the thought: "I have to use porn right now." crept into my mind.

Of course I tried to counter it by thinking: "NO. I can't do porn. Not again", and initially I did manage to stop myself with it, but then, an hour later the addicted part of my mind attacked me again: "Oh come on. Porn is no big deal. What harm it can do?" I again said "NO", and to that it replied 'Someday. Someday." It didn't take much time before I started worrying about whether or not I'll relapse. "Will I relapse?" "How can I be sure I won't relapse?" I even used a pendulum and tarot reading to 'predict' that I won't relapse in order to calm myself down. It didn't work. My worrying just increased. I ruminated and ruminated: "Oh maybe using porn is not so bad. I mean I struggle with it so "Maybe it was better when I was addicted to porn, I at least didn't have to struggle that much." In that moment, I knew I couldn't stand another second of that kind of pressure, and my mind again said: "Maybe you'd feel better if you'd masturbate to weight gain porn. Come on just embrace your sexuality, what's wrong with using porn? Everyone does it." At that time, while struggling with my uncertainty, I finally cracked and yet again masturbated, this time to amputee porn. In that moment, all uncertainty washed away. I had room to breathe. The problem is that that space of uncertainty disappeared very quickly. The relief from uncertainty that I got from using porn was very short-lived and I would come back to my struggle again and again. This fueled my addiction for a long time.

YOUR MISTAKES DON'T EQUAL THE PAST.

For every addict, the past is a source of constant regret. I can't tell you how many times I've beaten myself up. Here are some of the things I used to constantly ruminate about:

- "I've destroyed my sexuality with my masturbation habits."
- "Oh why did I do this?"
- "I'll never be able to have a functional relationship."
- "Why did I ever get into extreme fetish porn. How could I ever think this was a good idea?"
- "It was my fault. I was overconfident. I should have never touched porn."

But no matter where you are in life and with your addiction, you can make your own story. You can live a rich and meaningful life. You'll be able to say: "yes, that life, that kind of living, is mine, and I am grateful to have it."

The more I was preoccupied with my past or future. The less effective I was in the present.

PAIN IS INEVITABLE.

You'll experience unpleasant things. It's a given. But when you try to escape the pain of life by making a fist and tensing up, it's hard to experience the pleasures of life. When your hands are covering your eyes you can't see a flower or a beautiful sunset or see anything that's available to you. We're evolutionary predisposed to hiding, and running. It's the easiest way to 'survive'. For this reason it's a very scary thing to let go of hiding, fighting and running.

One of the first things you see once you'll stop hiding is the damage that hiding has brought upon you. When we're hiding, there are two things we really pay attention to: the thing we're escaping from and the thing that we see as 'the way out'. If you were in a building escaping from a monster you'd be most aware of the monster and the exit. You'd probably completely ignore all the finer details of the store, such as the color of the walls, or what other people are doing in that building.

Running from your past or future works the same way. When you're run, hide or fight you become less aware of your life in the present moment.

NO OTHER LIVING THINGS SUFFERS LIKE A HUMAN.

What is the difference between a dog and a human? When you kick a dog out into the rain and then let him back in he'll dry himself up and continue being happy as he was before the event. When you kick a human into the rain and let him back he'll go over what led up to it, rage about how unfairly he was treated, and plot revenge on the person who threw him out.

PURE PAIN VS DIRTY PAIN

If you think about it, zebras and rabbits have it far worse than us. They have to fight for their lives every day, and every day they live in a pretty uncomfortable environment. They sleep on grass, rocks, and very often get scraped and bruised while walking. They experience a lot of pain, and yet they don't suffer. The difference between their pain and our pain is that their pain is clean our pain is dirty.

Clean pain is pain free from resistance, judgments and thoughts about it. It's just pain as it is experienced in the present moment, without anything thinking added to it. It's painful, but it doesn't create suffering.

On the other hand, dirty pain is pain that's infused with our own judgments and our own thoughts about the situation. When someone kicks you in the nuts you don't only experience the pain but you also create a story behind it such as: "Damn it. I got kicked in the nuts. Life is so unfair" and you try to resist the pain. You think to yourself "I shouldn't feel this pain. This is wrong" and as such you strengthen your pain, and maybe even try to escape from it by masturbating to porn.

SUFFERING HAPPENS ALL THE TIME FOR HUMANS

We humans don't just suffer, suffering happens all the time for us. We suffer because we have suffered in the past, and we suffer because we might suffer in the future. No matter what kind of a good thing happens to us, there's always something better that might have happened to us. There's always a "before" we wish we could go back to or an "after" we wish we got and the present is always "later". "After this" "After that". The day of contentment is always tomorrow. But that tomorrow never comes. Only the present moment is real.

There's an alternative to waiting and searching for the right circumstance. What if you could act in a way that would fulfill you no matter how badly you felt and no matter how your life is at this moment? That's the promise of the NoPorn plan. But that promise is something you'd have to work on. It's the skill of mindfulness, and just like every skill. The skill to be mindfully in the present is a skill that has to be trained.

IF you want presence to be available in hard-risk situations, such as the situations when you're most likely to relapse on porn, you'll have to train it very well. This is why this book will have a lot of meditation exercises, and you'll be expected to do all of them.

OUR MINDS HAVE EVOLVED TO SUFFER.

Our brains have evolved to make running and hiding seem like the best course of action. That is the case in the wild for prey. A monkey can either fight or run. If it 'accepts' and tries to befriend a tiger, it will die.

So when we're faced with uncomfortable situations, we also try to run and hide. Many of us use porn, drugs and alcohol to hide from our triggers and our uncomfortable, painful life experiences.

Our brains have also learned to hate uncertainty. Uncertainty meant a danger was afoot. Uncertainty meant you could be killed at any moment. The problem is that while we want the world to sit still and behave so we'll feel safe, life won't work this way. It's full of change and uncertainty.

Similarly our brains have evolved to always picture a "better tomorrow" in order for us to search for a place with no lions and predators. Contentment was something very dangerous to our ancestors. When a monkey stopped running and struggling, it was quickly eaten by a tiger.

Our minds are problem-solving mechanisms that aim to reach perfection. The problem with this is this creates a situation where there always will be a 'better than now' and if we'll allow ourselves to be taken over by our mind, we'll be never be content in our life, as our minds are not built for peace. They are built for struggle and they are built to avoid suffering.

The problem is that suffering is inevitable. This Buddhist parable illustrates this point perfectly:

A woman whose son has died came to the Buddha and she asked him to revive her child. He said he'd be able to do so, but only if she could give him a mustard seed from a garden of a family that never suffered loss or pain in their lives. The woman struggled to find such a family or such a person. But she failed.

Pain is an inevitable part of human experience. The trick behind living a productive and fulfilling life is to learn how to deal with pain and ACT in a value-driven way. This is also the secret to beating porn addiction, which you'll learn in this book.

Our brains have also evolved to HATE change because change always brings uncertainty. When you try to change (Wilson & DuFrene, 2012) your brains will think: "I might live a shitty life. But it's my shitty life. It's familiar. It might not be pleasant. But it's safe. How do I know it? I'm alive and deep down that's all I care about."

The primitive part of your brain doesn't really care about your values, achievement, productivity or even pleasure. Our brains were not designed for us to be happy. They were designed for us to survive. From the perspective of our brain, everything that we habitually do is 'good enough' as we're not in an immediate risk of dying, and as such we have to be doing something right, and 'it's a risk to change a 'good thing'.

As a recovering addict, you'll have to face a LOT of uncertainty and a lot of change. But we'll help you to learn how to bypass the natural impulse to escape and hide from life by learning mindfulness skills, and building your mindfulness muscles. Among other things, you'll learn to make friends with uncertainty.

Why do we have to make friends with uncertainty? Because everything in life that's worth doing carries with itself at least a bit of uncertainty:

- Adopting a new exercise schedule - Uncertainty.
- Changing your diet - Uncertainty.

- **Starting a new job - Uncertainty.**
- **Going to College - Uncertainty.**
- **Quitting an addiction - Uncertainty.**
- **Dating - Uncertainty.**

Everything in life that is worth doing involves uncertainty. Even with my currently relationship with my significant other, she and I both had to overcome uncertainty with transitioning from a long distance online relationship to her living with me in person as independent autistic adults. This in itself is a long story, but it all started September 12, 2013. She and I met online for the first time on a dating page for adult autistic people. From that day we really clicked, no pun intended, and every day we talked to one another and fell a bit more in love. However it was not as simple as that, she was in a very dysfunctional home and struggling with alcoholism and depression two years after graduating from University of Michigan in Ann Arbor with her BA, and I was struggling myself with porn addiction and my own personal and family issues. To complicate things further, she lived in Michigan and I in Poland. December 2013 she left her relatives behind and went homeless to Ann Arbor from Flint. From a distance I helped her make craiglist ads, cleaning for room and board. After she left the local shelter she was employed for room and board as a direct care worker in Ann Arbor and she and I stayed in contact online daily through Skype and Facebook.

Those seven months had some deep lows, including but not limited to myself having a suicide attempt March of 2014, and various issues here and there with her employment and mother harassing her.

Somehow though, she was able to save money from odds and ends and I was able to set things up on my end, and in August of 2014, she flew to Poland to be with me.

After 11 months of massive uncertainty and turmoil, we finally got to be together in a functional, loving, and sober relationship and make this program you are going through today.

The meditations and exercises found in this book will teach you how to become friends with uncertainty so that you can more easily change your life into exactly the life you want.

CAN YOU BECOME A HERO?

In modern media, a hero is portrayed as someone with a superpower and some skill, which he or her uses to effortlessly accomplish all the things he wants and help others in the process. But what makes a real hero? What's the one factor that connects Gandhi, Martin Luther King Jr., and everyone else we historically see as a hero?

They simply faced the facts of life and even though life and people were needlessly cruel during those moments of time, they chose to act in accordance with their values, even if they had to embrace a lot of suffering to do so.

You don't need a magic sword or laser-eyes to be a true hero, you just need to act in accordance with your values, no matter how painful life gets.

1. Now I would like you to write down a list of issues that are psychologically difficult for you.

We want a list of psychological issues. "My wife" Is not correct. "Getting frustrated with my wife" is correct. Include any of your thoughts, feelings, memories, bodily sensations, habits or behavioral predispositions that may distress you. Just write anything that causes you pain.

2. Do you sense some kind of pattern? Do you generally find that you suffered in the long term as a result of avoidance?

3. How did you avoid them?

4. How long has each of these issues been a problem for you?

Simply copy the list you've written in the previous answer, and next to each problem write how long it's been a problem to you

5. Name a few thoughts and situations you've avoided.

6. Now I would like to group the issues you've identified in the previous question in pairs. Write down issues that might be related to one another in pairs.

For example if you wrote 'self-criticism' and depression. Write Depression/Self-criticism. This will allow you to see how your mental issues are interconnected.

7. Now I would like you to rank these problems in terms of the impact they had in your life. Write and number them from the most problematic to least problematic issues

From now on we'll refer to this list in the NoPorn plan as your 'suffering inventory'.

8. What happened immediately as a result of your avoidance?

9. What negative consequences happened eventually as a result of your avoidance?

In the next chapter we'll dwell more deeply into mindfulness and how you can use it to quit porn.

[6]

On Mindfulness and How It Can Help You Beat Your Sex and Porn Addiction

WE SUFFER WHEN WE TRY TO CONTROL WHAT WE CAN'T control. I also have tried to control things I couldn't control.

I have many personal stories with this as well. I not only 'fought' with my anxiety and depression, but I also fought with my chronic pain. My fight never amounted to anything. I still experience chronic pain to this day, my avoidance of it just kept me from exercising as often as I ought to and living my life as actively as I should. I even often used porn as a means of controlling my chronic pain and anxiety. I often masturbated to escape my feelings and internal sensation. While recovering from porn addiction, I sometimes relapsed in an attempt to control the strong feelings of sexual tension that I experienced in the first days of being porn free.

True acceptance in the form of mindfulness allows you to experience not only physical and emotional pain without being engulfed by it, but also your thoughts.

Most people are controlled by their thoughts. Not so long ago, whenever the addicted part of my brain would say "DO PORN", I would instantly identify with that thought and do exactly as it told me to, almost automatically. It was only after hours of learning the tools of mindfulness, where I would sit and become aware of what was moving inside my mind, and how to not allow these experiences to build up into the addictive behavior of Pornography

More often than not, I'm now able to hear the addicted part of my brain say "MASTURBATE TO PORN NOW! YOU CAN'T HANDLE LIFE AS IT IS!" I notice it, and then just move my attention to something more productive and move on with my life. You'll learn these skills more in the next lessons, but right now I want you to become aware of them.

I want to think of all the things you're doing to escape the urges to do porn and to escape your sexual and other feelings keeps you from living a valued life. Think of the time you spent watching porn, trying to control the urge to masturbate and struggling to manage the effects of extensive masturbation and porn use.

First, it's important to realize that watching porn and escaping sexual thoughts work only in the short term. If you happen to work as a programmer, you cannot escape all of your triggers. You'll sooner or later will have to work at a computer, which will trigger you eventually.

That's why the ultimate goal of therapy is not to eliminate all triggers from your life (although we'll try to limit them as much as possible) but to teach you how you can experience the urge to watch porn/masturbate without acting on it. (Harris, 2009)

Pain hurts. But it doesn't have to constrain our behavior. We can act in an optimal way no matter how terrible we feel. We very often focus on our pain and make our lives revolve around our anxiety and depression. Sometimes to the extent of getting a useless BSC in psychology as I did. One way to get over this unproductive belief that "I need to feel great in order to be great" is to imagine that someone has waved a magic wand over you and all of your emotional pain has vanished. What would you do? What would you want your life to be about?

HOW THE TRADITIONAL PROBLEM SOLVING MENTALITY CREATES PROBLEMS

Mental problems happen when we try to use the same strategies that are used in solving problems in the outside world to solve problems in our inner world, within us.

Let's now look at how we'd solve external problems by looking at how we'd react if we smelt gas in the kitchen:

- We'd recognize there's something wrong by detecting a strange smell.
- We'd identify the cause by noticing that the odor is gas from the stove and that one of the knobs isn't completely turned off.
- We'd anticipate that the house would probably explode if nothing gets done.
- We'd determine what should be done and do it. In this case we would turn the gas knob off.
- Then we'd evaluate whether it worked by comparing the outcome to the expected outcome. In this case, we would wait to see if the odor dissipates.
- Then we will determine what we learned and figure out how to handle similar problems in the future.

Now look all of these steps and think: How could they lead to suffering or psychological inflexibility if we would attempt to use them for internal problems?

For example, if we applied step 2: "Identifying a cause", to internal problems, could it be harmful if it shows up in the form of attributing blame or responsibility? ("It was my fault" or "You should have known better").

Likewise, apply step 3 to solve internal problems this might result in worrying. ("I know I need to do this, but what if ...?")

Step 4: "Determining what should be done and doing it", requires that we access an internal rule. But when we deal with internal problems trying to adhere to such rules, this creates thought patterns which include "should's" and "must's" which have been identified as the main cause of psychological problems by Cognitive Behavioral Therapy (Specifically Rational Emotive Behavioral Therapy)(Ellis & Ellis, 2011). But even if you think about this using common sense, a strict adherence to mental rules can lead to rigidity.

If we try to apply step 5 to internal events, this might result in a negative view of oneself because we'll constantly perform below our standard. ("Why I can't just stop being this way? or "I'm a loser, and most people probably think so too.")

And finally if we try to apply our judgments and evaluations into our internal landscape, this might lead to the creation of a negative self-image and viewing the world as harmful and limiting ("I should just stop trying", "Maybe if I stop caring, I won't get hurt again" or "That's how people are, so why should I bother getting close to anyone?")

So as you can see, it can lead to problems when we apply strategies that work for external problems to internal problems.

Let's now see what happens when we try to 'control' a thought and an urge. What if what you're doing with these thoughts, memories, and feelings is like fighting with a ball in a pool? You don't like these things. You don't want them, and you want them out of your life. So you try to push the ball under the water and out of your consciousness. However, the ball keeps popping back up to the surface, so you have to keep pushing it down or holding it under the water. Struggling with the ball in this way keeps it close to you, and it's tiring and futile. If you were to let go of the ball, it would pop up and float on the surface near you, and you probably wouldn't like it. But if you let it float there for a while without grabbing it, it could eventually drift away to the other side of the pool. And even if it didn't, at least you'd be able to use your arms and enjoy your swim, rather than spending your time fighting.

Here's another metaphor that illustrates the effect of trying to manage your emotions and urges through control:

Picture your life as a room. One day you notice that a pipe in the ceiling has started to leak. The messes the water creates as well as the sound of the falling drops makes you nervous and you want get rid of it. So you repair the leak with a length of duct tape and mop the water, your peace of mind is back--until the water finds its way through the tape and the dripping sound and the water mess is back: So you put another length of tape around the first repair and things are back in order again. Of course the peace and quiet doesn't last very long. You have to fix the leak again and again. That's not a big problem since duct tape is pretty cheap and you always manage to keep a spare roll handy. This goes on for months or even years until one day you notice that these big clumsy repairs are slowly filling the room, leaving less and less space for you to live in and only makes things worse by spreading even more water everywhere.

Living with openness to your experience takes practice, just like being comfortable with uncertainty takes practice. This is why you'll meditate for about an hour a day to develop this and other mindfulness skills that we'll be given to you here, that not only will help you break free from your porn addiction but they'll also help you lead a more productive life. Some meditations will work better for you than others. That's why I'll show you another mindfulness meditation called the body scan exercise.

This exercise will teach you how to get into your body and at will turn from your thoughts (not just pornographic thoughts, but any counterproductive thoughts) into the body. When you turn yourself in the body you're automatically put into the present moment, which will allow you to optimally react to your current situation. This exercise teaches you this skill. It's one of the few exercises in the book that we recommend you practice repeatedly, as it's less about teaching you concept but instead directly teaches you a skill. A mindfulness skill. The more you practice it the stronger your 'mindfulness muscle' will become.

EXERCISE:

1. What do I do to control the urges to watch porn and/or masturbate to porn? (E.g. masturbate to porn, avoid situations that make me have sexual thoughts, etc.)

2. How well do these strategies work in the short term? What about long term? Does the urge to watch porn usually comes back?

3. What are the costs or disadvantages of these strategies?

4. Is my struggle with these urges getting greater or less over the months and years? Am I succeeding or falling more and more behind?

6. If someone has waved a magic wand over you and all of your anxiety, depression, and other emotional pain just vanished, what would you do?

7. What would you want your life to be about?

8. How has your current psychological struggle interfered with your goals and aspirations?

9. Complete this sentence with every emotion from your suffering inventory: If ____ was not such a problem for me. I would...

We would like you to fill in the blank lines in the sentences below, but first let us describe how to do that. Take an item from your suffering inventory you've completed in the previous lesson. It could be any item, but it might be best to start with an item high on your list and connected to other items. This is probably an issue that greatly inhibits your life. Go ahead and fill in your problem, but don't fill in what you would do if it were gone.

Now, think about what you would do if that pain were suddenly lifted. The point of this exercise is not to think about what you might like to do on a given day if your problems weren't plaguing you. The idea isn't to celebrate by saying, "My depression is gone, and I'm going to Disneyland!" The point is to think more broadly about how your life course would change if your constant struggle with emotional pain was no longer an issue. Don't worry if you think that you don't have a good grip on this yet. We will do a lot more work with this later in the NoPorn Plan when we'll discuss your values.

Here are a few examples of what I want you to write:

• If I didn't have so much anxiety, I would be able to get the job I want.

• If anger wasn't such a problem for me, I would have fewer problems at work.

• If I didn't have such a strong feeling of depression, I would work harder at my job, and I would try to find a job that I always wanted.

10. Do the same here: If I didn't have ____ I would...

11. Do you remember the steps we need to take to solve external problems? Name a few ways how each of these steps could create suffering.

You can refer to the examples given in the lesson.

12. See if you can effectively control your thoughts.

For the next few seconds, I'd like you to not think about a puppy. You can think about anything else other than a puppy. If thoughts of a cute little puppy that wags his tail and jumps on you to lick your face come up, go ahead and push those thoughts away and don't think about them. You can think about anything else, but whatever you do, don't think about a puppy. Do this for 4 minutes. Have you successfully been able not to think about a puppy? What strategies have you used to not think about a puppy? How effective were they?

BODY SCAN MEDIATION:

Find a friend to read it to you. Alternatively you can get a recorded version of this meditation in my website at http://nopornplan.com. You will also get a free comic book that will expand on the things you're learning in this book.

In this exercise, you'll scan your body from head to toe, noticing whatever sensations might be there. The aim is to observe these sensations without judging them, trying to change them or push them away.

If you notice tension or discomfort in your body, simply allow it to be there. Don't try to change it. Don't try to escape from it. Simply observe it. If your mind starts judging it or commenting on it, simply let these thoughts pass like cars on the road.

If you find your mind wandering, creating judgment, ideas, or thoughts, simply let that mind chatter come and go like birds flying across the window outside, then gently bring your attention back to the exercise. This exercise is essentially the equivalent of pushups for your mindfulness muscles and you'll do well to repeat it from time to time to strengthen them.

Either sit down or lie down on some surface and allow your eyes to close, letting your hands lay on the sides of your body. Your legs should be uncrossed. For the next few minutes, remind yourself that during this time there's nothing you have to do, and no one you have to please. This is your time. Your time to be present here and now, and to notice what's happening in this moment with an attitude of openness and curiosity.

Aim to cultivate the attitude of a curious scientist, as you become open to your experience right here, right now.

Pause

When you're ready bring your attention to the physical sensations in your abdomen, becoming aware of the sensations as you breathe in and exhale out. Take a few minutes to feel the changing sensations, how the inhaling feels different than the exhaling.

Pause

Now move your attention to your feet, noticing what sensations are in both feet when the attention arrives here. Notice the sensations in the toes.

Notice the sensations in the soles of your feet.

The heels.

Top of the feet

What's here right now?

If there are no sensations simply register a blank. If they are subtle notice it regardless. There's nothing you should or should not feel. What you experience is the correct experience.

Pause

Now take a breath in and out, and then move your attention to the ankles. What sensations are there? Whatever sensations you notice, allow them to be there. Just let them be. Don't try to change anything. You don't have to like or want these sensations or approve of them in any way. All you need to do is observe them without struggling.

From time to time your attention will become distracted by thoughts or feelings. Each time that happens, take a split second to note what distracted you and bring your attention back to the body. And no matter how often your attention wanders. Whether it's a few or a thousand times. Just notice what distracted you and gently bring your attention back to the body. There's no need to be frustrated or disappointed when this happens. We expect your attention to wander. It's part of being human. And each time you bring your attention back to where you want it to be, you're training your mindfulness muscles.

Pause

Now take yet another breath and on the outbreath move your attention to the lower legs. What sensations do you feel in them?

Pause

Notice any sense of contact with whatever you're resting on. Welcome any sensation that might arise.

Pause

Now take another deep breath and as you breathe out, move your attention to the knees. Don't think about the knees, but sense directly what they experience right now. Notice what sensations change, and what sensations stay the same.

Pause

If your mind starts judging. criticizing, commenting, analyzing, just let those thoughts come and go. And bring your attention back to the sensations in this part of your body.

Pause

Now take another deep breath and as you breathe out, move your attention to your thighs. What do you feel there? It could be the sensation of contact with your clothes. It could be a pulsation. It could be anything. Whatever it is. Allow yourself to welcome it in.

During this exercise your mind will wander away from your body. This is completely normal. When you notice it, acknowledge it, and then return your attention back to your body.

Pause

Now take another deep breath and as you breathe out, move your attention to the hips and pelvis. The hip to the right. The hip to the left, and the whole base of the pelvis and the organs in this region.

Pause

Now take another deep breath and as you breathe out, move your attention to the lower back. And now as you breathe in, expand your awareness to take in the middle of the back.

Pause

And now on another breath, expand your awareness to take in the upper back and the rest of your back, until you are fully aware of your entire back, noticing any sensations that might arise in it.

Pause

Now take another breath, and as you exhale move your attention to the front of your body, to the lower abdomen. Notice the sensations there as your attention moves into this area of your body.

Pause

From time to time, feelings of boredom or restlessness might come up. When this happens know that nothing's gone wrong. Simply notice these feelings and distractions and acknowledge them. Notice how they're affecting your body, and without judging yourself in any way move your attention back to the lower abdomen.

Pause

Now take a deep breath and on the outbreath move your attention to the chest. Notice what sensations you experience in your chest.

Pause

Now take a deeper breath into the chest. As you let go of the breath let go of your attention on the chest and move your attention to both of your hands and arms. Focus on them.

Pause

Now take a breath and on the outbreath move your attention from the arms to your shoulders and neck. What sensations are here? Whatever they are. Allow them to be exactly as they are.

Pause

Take another deep breath. And on the outbreath move your attention to your head and face. Notice your chin, your mouth, your lips, the surface of the nose, the cheeks, the sides of the face and the ears, the eyes, the eyelids, the eyebrows, the temples, and the space between the eyebrows. The forehead, and the temples, and the scalp.

Now expand your awareness to take in your whole face, and just allow the sensations in it to be as they are.

Now expand your awareness further to envelope your whole body, and just allow the sensations you feel in it to be exactly as they are. When you'll find your attention wandering move your attention back to the sensations in your body. Allow your body to be just as it is. Allow yourself to be just as you are. Complete as you are, resting in awareness.

WHAT IS WILLINGNESS?

Willingness is a very important mindfulness skill. Willingness is also called acceptance. (They are synonymous) In the context of acceptance and commitment therapy (on which the NoPorn Plan is based on) acceptance is the ability to be present with what you think and feel without trying to suppress it or 'get rid of it'. It's simply the willingness to experience life as it is in the moment, no matter how painful it is. (Hayes & Smith, 2005). It's not approving, wanting, or liking it, nor will acceptance change it. It's simply the ability to face life as it is. Many New Age authors claim that if you "allow life to be as it is" it will somehow magically change and everything will be better. (Byrne, 2006) Similarly, many new age authors claim that if you just accept your feelings that will somehow 'discharge' them and you'll be happy. These people tell you that because it's extremely hard to sell someone 'feeling his feelings' without the promise that negative feelings and circumstances will go away, and at the same time most of the new age courses that say that your problems will 'go away' if you 'do a mental technique' know that the kind of people who buy such courses won't even bother to do a mental exercise since they expect things to happen automatically. Every successful person who overcame real problems faced them didn't approve of them, want them or like them. They simply acknowledged that they exist, and choose to act in a way that's congruent with their values. This is the essence of acceptance and commitment therapy. I've mentioned in previous lessons, training mindfulness through meditation is the key to overcoming porn addiction. Mindfulness is a skill that is composed of acceptance. When you're mindfully aware you consider, notice, and observe. I stress again, when you accept something it does not mean you approve of it, like it or want it.

For example, If you get sick with the flu, you can accept and experience the uncomfortable feelings in your nose as they happen in that moment, and your thoughts about the flu, without liking or wanting the illness. Acceptance doesn't mean that you 'want or like something', it means that when a particular experience arises, you simply acknowledge it and choose to be present with it and experience it and not force a change in that moment. Your acceptance of these things will not get rid of them, but it will turn dirty pain into clean pain. Acceptance in the therapeutic sense of the word is defined as being able to feel what you feel, think what you think, and see and hear what you see and hear, even if it's unpleasant or painful. It's about being intentionally open to everything and anything you experience in your present moment awareness. (Hayes & Smith, 2005)

It's What Distinguishes Meditation from Rumination

Acceptance is also the main quality that differentiates meditation and mindfulness from rumination. When you're mindful, you're aware of your thoughts but you don't resist them. Instead you just allow yourself to experience them without being taken away by them. The technical term for being 'taken away' by your thoughts and feelings is Fusion. The ability to not be taken away by them, which is fostered by acceptance, is called Defusion. (Hayes & Smith, 2005). If you think about it, you cannot change an experience in the moment you're experiencing it. Let's say that I kick you in the teeth, and as result you'll feeling ball the moment I did it, whether you like it or not and you can't do anything about it. The pain will not subside more if you 'don't like it' as opposed to 'liking it'. Whether you decide to kick my teeth afterwards is a conscious cognitive choice related to your values.

It also doesn't mean that your judgments will go away. If you're sick, you'll most likely have thoughts like "this is terrible" or "why is this happening to me?" You'd also experience similar thoughts if someone kicked you in the teeth. Part of healthy acceptance is noting and accepting your resistance to the experience and your automatic judgments about the experience.

Again, acceptance also is not resignation. Resignation is about giving up something, while acceptance is about opening up to experiences.

In Many Ways, Acceptance Is Like Eating an Apple

Acceptance is like eating an apple. One reason for eating an apple could be because you're trying to eat healthier, so you're trying to stay away from things that are "bad" for you. So instead of your usual snack, let's say a chocolate cupcake, you tell yourself you'll have an apple. You may "choose" an apple, but what will it be like to eat that apple? As you eat it, you start comparing it to the cupcake. With each bite, you're thinking about how the apple isn't as sweet, fudgy, or soft as the cupcake. Then, when you're done, you eat the cupcake anyway. What we're talking about here is another way to eat an apple: allowing the apple to be an apple, rather than needing or wanting it to be something it's not and never will be. Noticing the crispiness of each bite, the juiciness, and the sweetness for what it is and not for what it isn't – a cupcake

I HAD A PROBLEM WITH UNDERSTANDING ACCEPTANCE TOO

Honestly, I had a major problem with acceptance. I had suffered from PTSD and panic attacks for years as a kid and I grew up in a fairly abusive household with an alcoholic father, a neglectful mother, and antagonistic relatives and community. So for most of my life, I tried to escape reality and existence as it was. This was one of the main factors that drove me to use pornography as much as I once did. For me, it was a form of escape. I know now that if I learned to accept reality using the meditations and techniques I am sharing with you, my addiction would have never spiraled to the extent it did and I would have never had the problems I had.

For most of my life, I practiced the opposite of acceptance. I religiously practiced avoidance because I thought it was the only thing that would allow me even a speck of happiness. For most of my life I wanted nothing more than to escape from my reality into something else. Porn seemed like the strongest and most tangible form of escape.

I used porn as an escape from the fact that I did not have any friends, from the fact that I did badly at school and from the fact that I felt like a loser. Every proactive attempt at helping me brought with it other negative feelings. Studying felt boring, exercising felt tedious, approaching people felt scary.

Back then, I simply lacked the mindfulness required to face any of these feelings. This wasn't a 'fault' thing, it was simply an untrained muscle, and I didn't have the tools to train it. I was no more 'faulty' for being the way I was than for the fact I was weak when I didn't have access to the gym or even dumbbells. I now know my life would have been completely different if I had the tools I'm teaching in this program that would allow me to train mindfulness so I could have faced my issues instead of escaping from them.

Because the truth is <u>no one really gets through life without getting hurt</u>. Pain is inevitable and you'll always experience it. Trying to escape from it through porn, drugs, video games or anything else just makes things worse. Ruminating on your failures does the same.

<u>In short acceptance is all about embracing what is and what life offers. It's all about saying "yes" to life exactly how it is.</u> The important thing to notice right now is that acceptance is not a concept. It's a skill to be learned. You'll learn this skill through a daily meditation practice. This skill will allow you to be unmoved by any urges to masturbate to porn and it will loosen the grip your addiction has on you.

EXERCISE:

1. Complete the following sentences:
   - The thoughts I'd most like to get rid of are:
   - The feelings I'd most like to get rid of are:
   - The sensations I'd most like to get rid of are
   - The memories I'd most like to get rid of are:

2. Next, take a few minutes to write a list of the things you've tried in order to get rid of these things. Try to remember every strategy you've ever used.

Strategies such as:

Distraction- List everything you used to distract yourself from negative feelings, memories or thoughts.

Opting out - List all the activities, interests, events, people or places that you have avoided and all the opportunities you have missed out on, because you did not feel good or wanted to avoid feeling bad.

Thought strategies. List all the ways in which you have tried used thinking to escape from painful thoughts and feelings. Tick any of the following and write in any others:

- **Worrying**
- **Fantasizing about the future**
- **Dwelling on the past**
- **Imaging escape scenarios**
- **Imaging revenge scenarios**
- **Imaging suicide scenarios**
- **Thinking 'It's not fair...'**
- **Thinking 'If only...'**
- **Blaming yourself, others and the world**
- **Talking to yourself, either logically negatively or even positively**
- **Analyzing yourself. (Trying to figure out why you are like this)**
- **Analyzing the situation (trying to figure out why this happened)**
- **Analyzing others (trying to figure out why they are like this)**

3. Substances and other things you used to escape:
Try to list all of the substances and addictive things you've used to make yourself feel better. Including drugs, foods, drinks, porn, gambling, video games, the internet, movies, masturbating.

4. Or anything else?
Write down anything else you can think of that you've used to make yourself feel better when painful feelings showed up.

5. Once you've done all that. Go through this list and ask yourself

- Did this get rid of my painful thoughts and feelings in the long term?
- Did it bring me closer to a rich, full, and meaningful life?
- If the answer to question 2 is 'no' then what did this cost you in terms of time, energy, money, health, relationships and vitality?

ACCEPTANCE IS A PROCESS. IT'S NEVER CONSTANT.

Acceptance is something you have to practice moment by moment. It's not something you 'achieve' and 'master'. That's why it's crucial to accept the inevitable; resistance to life happens to even the most experienced mediators.

To give you a feeling of acceptance I would like you to practice a mindfulness exercise developed by Tara Brach called the "Yes Exercise." It will show you how you can say either Yes or No to every experience, and how it can influence your experience.

Have a friend read it to you. Alternatively you can get a recorded version of this meditation at http://nopornplan.com You will also get a comic that will expand on what you've learned here.

In this exercise, I'm going to ask you to avoid experiencing the sensations you have of your back against the chair you're sitting in. For the next two to three minutes, whenever you notice a sensation of your back against the chair, I want you to say no to those sensations. Notice the reactions.

Pause

Just say No. Resist the feeling of your back against your chair.

Pause

Notice the feeling of your skin touching your clothes. Say no to it. Notice the reaction.

Pause

Notice the sensation of touch on your skin. Say no to it. Resist it. What's the reaction?

Pause

Now I'd like you to notice any thoughts and emotions that might show up and also say NO to these thoughts and emotions. Notice the reaction.

Pause

Notice any thought that might come up, and resist it, as you might normally resist any unpleasant thought that comes your away. Do your hardest to resist it.

Pause

You might notice that the thoughts are getting louder the more you resist them. That's the natural outcome of resistance. Now notice another thought. And try to resist it

Pause

Now notice whatever might arise in your consciousness and say NO to it

Pause
Say no to it.
Pause
Resist it.

Okay, now I'd like to do the same exercise, except now instead of avoiding the sensations of your back against the chair, I'd like you to be willing to feel the those sensations, simply as sensations, whatever they may be, positive or negative: pain, discomfort, tingling, warmth, coolness, and so on. Whatever those sensations are, I'd like you to say yes to them.
Pause
Just say yes to them.
Pause
Just notice whatever arises in your consciousness and say yes to it. Allow them to be as they are.
Pause
Say yes to it.
Pause
Yes, could you just allow it to be as it is?
And now as you stop this exercise. Could you just see what happens when you say yes, to everything that you experience? Open your eyes and see if you can continue this attitude of yes, throughout the day.

WHAT ACCEPTANCE IS NOT

I have found that its always helpful to explain a concept by explaining what it is not. Let's now look at what acceptance is not.

ACCEPTANCE IS NOT RESIGNATION

Acceptance in the therapeutic sense of the word is not resignation or defeat, in fact the opposite is true. Change is empowered when you accept the present moment and embrace the uncomfortable moments that will inevitably occur during the process of change. For example let's take someone in an abusive situation. Acceptance would be helpful in this situation, but it wouldn't be acceptance of the abuse. It would mean accepting the facts, such as the fact that if nothing is done about the abuse, it will continue. It would mean acknowledging and becoming aware of the painful reality of your current situation. It would mean that you'd have to face your fears and the truth of your unworkable relationship. But it would not mean giving in.

Acceptance is all about accepting the facts. Accepting reality.

ACCEPTANCE IS NOT FAILURE

Acceptance is not an admission of failure. It's just a realization that a particular strategy cannot work. Acceptance is very related to workability. Acceptance is all about clearly seeing what works and what doesn't and abandoning the strategies that don't work. To actually take action to change, you need to accept that what you currently have is bad.

Acceptance is also not tolerance, although the distinction is not as clear. When you tolerate something, you want 'something out of it'; you want to 'feel the pain to get the prize'. Acceptance is an active process that suggests that there's something meaningful in every moment you can fully experience.

Acceptance is not a technique; it's a choice and a trained skill. It's not a matter of have to; it's a value-based leap. Feeling what one is feeling is not an end of itself- that's wallowing. Acceptance is not a trick designed to "accept something out of existence."

Willingness and acceptance have an all-or-nothing quality to it. You either face it or you don't. It's like jumping. But at the same time, willingness is not a desire to experience something

Let me now give you a metaphor that will illuminate the difference between being willing to have an experience (which is what acceptance as ACT understands it is) and wanting or desiring an experience:

Imagine yourself sitting on a plane for an overnight flight. You have the whole row to

yourself and you find comfort on the loneliness, all this space allows you now to stretch out and even get some sleep. Then, just before the cabin door is closed, a young couple comes on board with a crying baby; you begin to think, "The poor people who have to sit next to them all night!" Just as that thought crosses your mind, you see the couple moving toward you. They're seated next to you! You shuffle your stuff to make room for them, but in your head you're thinking, "No!" They smile and thank you for helping them get to their seats, and all the while their baby is screaming.

They try everything to soothe him. They try feeding him, and that just makes him

cry louder. They try his favorite toy, but he keeps screaming. What are your

options here? You can spend the next eight hours giving them dirty looks, scoffing at

their failed attempts to quiet their child, and letting them know that this kind of

behavior is absolutely unacceptable on a plane. Alternatively, you could join them in

trying to quiet the child: playing peekaboo, giving the child your phone to fiddle

with - doing anything to make the baby quiet. Or, you could choose to do what you would otherwise do on an overnight flight while taking in the sounds of that child as they

are and recognizing that the child is doing exactly what children do - Not wanting or

liking the sounds the child is making, but also not needing the sounds not to be there.

And all the while, you're also noticing that no matter how long the child cries, he

won't cry forever, and that wanting him to quiet down will never be what's needed to

make him quiet.

Let's now further illuminate the concept of acceptance by looking on a metaphor very commonly given in the course of Acceptance and Commitment Therapy.

How Acceptance Is Directly Related To Porn Addiction

The purpose of acceptance treatment is **NOT** to accept your porn use or your fetishes. It's to accept your **URGES** to use porn, **YOUR URGE** to masturbate to fetish porn.

The number 1 rule of all urges is:

The more you try to control them, the more you have them.

You can either accept your urges and take their power away, or you can fight them and resent them, raging war with yourself. When you're at war with yourself, you're at war with yourself forever until you chose to let go of the fight. Acceptance will not make you suffer less. Practicing acceptance doesn't make anything go away. It just stops it from unnecessarily growing.

That being said there's no guarantee that accepting an emotion will make it weaker. In fact it sometimes might make it stronger. It's not about making an emotion go away. You could be saying to yourself: "I don't know what will happen if I choose to just make room for my negative emotions and my urges. It could get worse; you never know. This seems risky."

I guess we could say that we know for sure what will happen if you keep fighting with this stuff. You'll probably keep getting the results you've been getting. Would you be willing to experiment with a different move and just see what happens?

You might think that "I first need to understand my problem before I can accept it"

Many people think that they first need to understand or get in touch with the 'deeper meaning' of a problem before they can be with it. This is simply not true. Allow me to illustrate that with yet another metaphor:

Cars are complicated and you might not know how they work. Do you know all the details about your car? Do you really have to figure out the intricate details of how a car internally works to drive it? Will understanding how the internal computer of a car works really help you drive back home from work??

This is parallel to trying to understand your feelings and thoughts when doing so won't help you move in a valued direction, and might even be a barrier

EXERCISE

In this mindfulness exercise you'll learn how to use willingness in order to better manage emotions. You'll be able to use this emotional mindfulness exercise each time you'll feel a negative emotion. By doing this you'll keep it from becoming a trigger, which in turn will keep you from relapsing to pornography. Have a friend read it to you. Alternatively you can get a recorded version of this exercise at http://nopornplan.com

In a previous exercise you experienced first-hand the difference between willingly experiencing your life and resisting it. This exercise is nothing more but a slightly more advanced version of the exercise you experienced previously.

Sitting quietly, close your eyes and take a few deep breaths. Bring to mind a current situation that elicits a manageable negative emotion. Get in touch with the memory of that experience. What is it about this situation that provokes the strongest feelings? You might see a particular scene in your mind, hear words that were spoken. Be especially aware of the feelings in your stomach, chest and throat.

In order to see firsthand what happens when you resist experience, begin by experimenting with saying no. As you connect with the pain you feel in the situation you have chosen, mentally direct a stream of no at the feelings. Say no to the negative emotions. Let the word carry the energy of no - Rejecting, pushing away what you are experiencing.

As you say no, notice what this resistance feels like in your body.

Pause

Do you feel tightness, pressure?

Pause

What happens to the painful feelings as you say no?

Pause

What happens to your heart?

Pause

Imagine what your life would be like if, for the next hours, weeks and months, you continued to move through the world with the thoughts and feelings of no.

Take a few deep breaths and let go by relaxing through the body, opening your eyes or shifting your posture a bit. Now take a few moments to call to mind again the painful situation you'd previously chosen, remembering the images, words, beliefs and feelings connected with it.

Pause

Now direct the word "yes" at your experience. Agree to the experience with yes.

Pause

Let the feelings float, held in the environment of yes. Even if there are waves of no -From the negative emotions that arise with the painful situation or even from doing this exercise- that's okay.

Pause

Let these natural reactions be received in the larger field of yes.

Pause

Yes to the pain.

Pause

Yes to the parts of us that want the pain to go away.

Pause

Yes to whatever thoughts or feelings arise

Pause

Notice your experience as you say yes. Is there softening, opening and movement in your body?

Pause

Is there more space and openness in your mind?

Pause

What happens to the unpleasantness as you say yes?

Pause

Does it get more intense?

Pause

Does it become more diffuse?

Pause

What happens to your heart as you say yes?

Pause

What would your experience be in the hours, weeks and months to come, if you could bring the spirit of yes to the inevitable challenges and sorrows of life?

Pause

Continue to sit now, releasing thoughts and resting in an alert, relaxed awareness. Let your intention be to say a gentle YES to whatever sensations, emotions, sounds or images may arise in your awareness.

Pause

As you open your eyes. See if you can keep this Yes attitude throughout your day.

EXERCISE

1. We are going to ask you to hold your breath. As you hold it follow the instructions listed below. Read them over a few times before you start. Don't start until you see the word start. Just read the following description.

When you do the exercise and the urge to breathe becomes stronger, we want you to do the following: Notice exactly where the urge to breathe begins and ends in your body. Locate exactly where you feel the urge to breathe.

See if you can allow that feeling to be precisely there and, at the same time, keep on holding your breath. Turn your willingness dial all the way up! Just feel the feeling and do not breathe... Think of this as a unique opportunity to feel something you rarely feel.

Notice any thoughts that come up, and gently thank your mind for the thought, without being controlled by that thought. Watch out for sneaky thoughts that can quickly lead to breathing before you decide to breathe. After all, who is in charge of your life? You or your mind? Notice other emotions that may emerge other than the urge to breathe. See if you can make room for those emotions, as well.

Survey your entire body and notice that, in addition to the urge to breathe, your body contains other sensations and continues to function.

Stay with the commitment to hold your breath as long as you can. As the urge to breathe becomes stronger, imagine that you are continuously creating that urge deliberately. Close your eyes and see if you can replicate this urge in your imagination, divorced from your body. With every pang in your chest, every worry you have about passing out, every instinct to breath, shift it from something unwelcome that is being visited upon you to something you are creating deliberately, just for the sake of feeling what that feels like.

This new urge is formally the same, but it is of your creation. Do you need to be threatened by your own creation?

Before beginning to hold your breath, list one or two other actions you might do during this exercise that might help you to be aware of all of your feelings, thoughts, sensations, and urges while you are holding fast to the goal of holding your breath. Write down only acceptance strategies, not experiential control or suppression strategies.

2. Read the description several times until you feel you completely understand the instructions. You are ready to see if it is possible to better control your behavior (holding your breath) by learning to accept and make room for your thoughts and feelings

Now START

Take a deep breath and hold it as long as you can. When you've finished write down how long you held it in your journal in seconds. You can assist yourself with a chronometer.

3. Describe your experience during this exercise.

4. Did the adversity of not breathing tend to come and go? When did it go up or down?

5. How did your mind try to persuade you to breathe before you really had to?

6. What was the sneakiest thing your mind did?

7. Do you see any possible implications this simple exercise might have for how your life has been going, especially in overcoming your porn addiction? If so, what do you see?

8. Now I want you to look back at the previous exercise in which we told you to hold your breath and check for how long you were able to hold your breath without using mindfulness and acceptance strategies. And compare it to the result you got when you held your breath with them. What was the difference? If you weren't able to see the application for this exercise for managing your porn addiction, does the comparison illuminate it a bit?

[7]

How to Take Control Over the Thoughts That Drive Your Sex and Porn Addiction

PROBLEMS ARISE WHEN we use our language and problem solving skills in instances when they're not helpful. If you ever listened to Osho or to any other old-time spiritual gurus, you might hear them say that "the mind is the enemy" or that "the secret to happiness is not thinking". There's some truth to this, but those gurus are too broad and not specific enough in their definition.

You feel anxiety and you try to 'figure it out' you try to find a way out. You'll try to escape these feelings, which will lead you into experiential avoidance. Your mind's attempt at solving the problem became the problem, because same things that work well in the external world and in school are very pathological in the internal world. (Hayes & Smith, 2005)

If you want to solve a math problem, you can do it easily with your mind and language abilities but if you don't like thinking about a past trauma and try to 'sweep it away' or 'understand it', you're just making it more central, more salient and more influential.

If we're afraid of rain we get an umbrella, but if we're afraid of rejection we'll avoid approaching women and avoid intimacy as a result.

Our judgments about the world are verbally acquired, and not based on direct experience. Our world and our social position in it are structured by our language, our story.

In a sense, the mind is not a thing but a collection of relational abilities, a collection of stories.

WE DON'T THINK IN FACTS. WE THINK IN STORIES.

This is why most people find movies and novels far more enjoyable than textbooks, and why fables have been used as a teaching tool for millennia.

Let's take the tale of the turtle and the hare. The slow moving steady turtle beat the overconfident hare. Through this story even a child can see the value of slow and steady progress, as opposed to overconfidence.

STORIES CAN LABEL US AND PIGEONHOLE US

In turn, as a rule we create stories about ourselves such as "Oh I'm a pervert" or "I'm a sinner". What kind of stories do you tell about yourself? Are you a sinner, are you a pervert?

The truth is that no one knows, and the greater truth behind this is that it doesn't matter at all. Unlike a fable, the stories we generally tell about ourselves do not have any value and don't contain any useful ideas.

ARE YOU A PERVERT?

It really depends on whom you ask. "Being a pervert" is a verb. It describes an action. Your action. In this moment -and the next and the next- you get to do something that re-frames the entire question.

Let's say that you tell yourself the story that you're the stupidest person in your class: do you do this to form an opinion of whether or not you're smart, or because you feel unable to learn something?

And what if your story is: "I'll never be able to quit masturbating to porn" or "I've masturbated for 15 years now and I'm going to masturbate till the day I die." Won't that story keep you from beating porn addiction?

The 'Conveyor Belt' mindfulness exercise will teach you how to let go of unproductive thoughts, and how to let them go. This will lower your stress, and will make you less likely to be triggered

CONVEYOR BELT

Remember you can get a recorded version of this meditation at http://nopornplan.com

This exercise is specifically designed to teach you the skill of letting thoughts come and go without getting caught up in them. Find a comfortable position. Either sitting up with your back straight or lying down flat on the floor.

Bring your attention to your breathing and observe your breath for a few seconds.

Pause

Imagine a moving black strip, a black strip that continuously moves past like a conveyor belt at a grocery store. Take each thought that pops up and place it onto that moving strip of black mass and let it move on by.

If your thought takes the form of a picture. Simply place it on the conveyor belt and let it float on by.

If your thought is made up of words, then put these words on the conveyor belt and let them move past.

That's all you need to do. No matter what the thought is. Even if it is a thought like "I can't do it. Or "This is stupid" simply take that thought, put it on the conveyor belt and let it move by.

No matter what the thought is, simply place it on the strip and let it float on by. If no thoughts or images are appearing simply let the conveyor belt move past. Each time a thought or an image appears simply put it on that strip and let it go by.

Long Pause for 2 Minutes

Now from time to time a thought will take up all of your attention and you'll lose track of this exercise. There's no need to beat yourself in the chest over this. It's normal and this is expected to happen. Whenever it happens simply note the thought that distracted you and put that thought on the conveyor belt and gently put your attention back to the exercise.

Long Pause for 2 minutes

Thoughts will repeatedly hook you in and you'll lose track of the exercise. This is normal. The moment you realize this has happened simply note the distraction, put it on the strip and carry on from where you left off.

1 Minute Pause

If you have the thought "I can't do it. I keep drifting away" Simply put it on the conveyor belt and carry on with the exercise

If you have the thought "this is boring" simply put it on the strip, let it pass, and carry on with the exercise

1 Minute Pause

And now bring your attention back to the breath. Follow the breath yet again. Take a moment to congratulate yourself for training this mindfulness skill. With regular practice you'll become far more proficient at letting your thoughts come and go, and you'll be able to let go of any thought about porn that might come up, no matter how seductive it might be. You'll also be able to let go of any negative thought no matter how painful it might be.

I recommend that you practice this exercise regularly, at least once per week. The more often you do it, the stronger your mindfulness muscles will become.

THE WILSON'S WAGER

What are the consequences of you assuming that the story is true or not true? If you assume that no one will ever love you and that you'll always be alone, you'll be exponentially more likely to use pornography, which in turn will make you more isolated and less likely to actually find someone in real life. I mean, if you assume that such story is true, why bother to conquer your porn addiction?

But what if you assume that you'll find love eventually? You'll probably approach people and although you might be rejected a few times, eventually you'll find someone who'll like you for what you are.

The Wilson's Wager created by Kelly G. Wilson, an associate professor of psychology at the University of Mississippi illustrates how having negative assumptions about our life has no real pragmatic benefit. (Wilson & DuFrene, 2012)

Assumption	Something extraordinary can happen	Something extraordinary can't happen
You assume Yes	Something extraordinary eventually happens!	You struggle and strive to no end
You assume No	You waste your life	Your life still stinks but you get to be 'right'

So as you can see. If you bet Yes, you either win or lose. But if you bet No, you either lose or lose. In this situation it's logical to bet yes, because No is always a losing bet.

You might want to quit using porn and you don't know if you can. Can you? We also don't know. And anyone who's honest with you about your addiction will give you that precise answer.

If you're in a bad situation right now due to your porn addiction, you might not be able to imagine the extent of something extraordinary happening in your life. What seems totally out of reach for you now: A steady job, a home of your own? It's likely that it all seems so out there that you don't dare let yourself even dream and wonder about it.

But thanks to Wilson's wager you now have a choice. You can choose to assume that something amazing can happen in your life. You can now do things that will make it more likely for it to happen. If you assume that something amazing can happen. It might. If you assume that it will never happen, it will never happen.

Alternatively you can assume that nothing good will happen in your life. When you do this and something good actual could happen in your life, you'll probably lose that chance at success.

Whenever we bet against ourselves it turns out we were right all along. This wager isn't designed to give you hope. It's designed for you to become a far savvier player in the game of life.

The truth is that all of our truths are given to us via correspondence: via language and symbols. They are models of the world. As such these models are not reality and since they're not reality you can swap them for something more productive. This philosophy is called <u>Functional Contextualism</u>. It says that if a belief/thought makes you function better, that determines whether or not it's true. As it did in the Wilson Wager. A story that supports you is functionally true. A story that distracts you from living a value-lead life is functionally false.

"If you follow what your story tells you to do here, what's likely to happen next?" or "How will you feel about that outcome if it does happen the way your story says it will? Is this the kind of life outcome you were hoping to get?"

EXERCISE

WHAT STORY IS YOUR MIND TELLING YOUR RIGHT NOW?

The human mind is like the world's greatest storyteller. It never shuts up. It's always got a story to tell, and more than anything else it just wants us to listen. It wants our full attention, and it will say anything to get our attention, even if it's painful or nasty or scary. And some of the stories it tells us are true. We call those facts. But most of the stories it tells us can't really be called facts. They're more like opinions, beliefs, ideas, attitudes, assumptions, judgments, predictions, and so forth. They're stories about how we see the world, what we want to do, what we think is right and wrong or fair and unfair, and so on. One of the things you and I want to do here is learn how to recognize when a story is helpful and when it isn't. So if you're willing to do an exercise, I'd like you to close your eyes and not say anything for about thirty seconds - just listen to the story your mind is telling you right now.

Now after a minute or two. Write down the story your mind has told you.

1.Name your stories

Identify your mind's favorite stories, and then give them names, such as the "loser!" story, or the "my life sucks!" story, or the "I can't do it!" story. Often there will be several variations on a theme. Write down your experience.

2.Thank your mind

This is a simple and effective defusion technique. When your mind starts coming up with those same old stories, simply be thankful. You could say to yourself (silently) things such as, "Thank you, Mind! How very informative!" or "Thanks for sharing!" or "Is that right? How fascinating!" or simply, "Thanks, Mind!"

When thanking your mind, don't do it sarcastically or aggressively. Do it with warmth and humor and with a genuine appreciation for the amazing storytelling ability of your mind. (You could also combine this technique with Naming the Story: "Ah yes, the 'I'm a failure' story. Thanks so much, Mind!")

COGNITIVE DEFUSION EXPLAINED

As you have learned in the first module of the NoPorn Plan, Cognitive Defusion is one of the mindfulness skills trained by Acceptance and Commitment Therapy. Cognitive Defusion is essentially buying into our thoughts, evaluations and beliefs. Fusion is most likely to occur in the following cognitive domains: judgments, rules, reasons, past future and self. We'll dissect and explain them in the following lessons, and give you exercises to train Cognitive Defusion. This will allow you to ACT in an optimal way even when your mind produces negative thoughts.

A simple example of cognitive defusion:

Let's say that you have the thought "Dating is scary, girls will think I'm stupid." you can see how fusion with this thought can result in not dating. While not going out and meeting women will allow you to avoid anxiety in the short-term, in the long-term it will make you lonely, more anxious and more prone to use porn to satisfy your sexual needs.

What if instead of buying into the thought: "Dating is scary, girls will think I'm stupid", you would simply watch it like you watch TV or a screen saver on a computer?

Let's now pick a more direct example. Let's take the thought "I have to use porn to relax". What do you think would happen if instead of buying into this thought, you'd simply see it as words that may or may not be true?

If buying into thoughts like:

- "I have to use porn right now",
- "I need to use porn",
- "I desire porn so much",
- "I can't live without porn. I need to use it",
- "I can't take this anymore I just want some release"

Causes you to use porn, simply observing these thoughts give you space to make a different choice more in alignment with your values.

Since fusion is something that we do automatically, it's very hard for us to understand Defusion without having a direct experience of it. You might have experienced some level of Cognitive Defusion while practicing the meditations you should have already practiced at this point in the book, but the following lessons will give you exercises specifically designed to allow you to understand and experience Cognitive Defusion. In In a moment I'll give you a meditation specifically designed to give you a direct experience of Cognitive Defusion.

IN COGNITIVE DEFUSION YOU BUY INTO YOUR JUDGMENTS

Language itself can throw us into interpersonal strife, and getting a sense of how this happens is key in learning how to limit self-inflicted suffering. This is especially the case when we evaluate people, moments, places, and ourselves. For language to work there has to be consistency or else we would not be able to communicate with one another. Also, the agreed label/description for a thing can't change until the thing itself changes completely.

For example: If I say "Here is a plain lamp," I can't in the next moment accurately call it a bear unless I somehow changed the lamp. I could paint a bear on it, or crudely make it into a bear sculpture; this however would not make it an actual bear but at least somewhat closer to being a bear. However, without a change in form, this is still just a plain lamp that can at best be a bear lamp. Just calling this lamp a bear does not make it a bear, conceptually.

Let's critique this lamp: I've said that this is a "plain" lamp, but a second opinion finds this lamp to be particularly feng shui. "Plain" and "feng shui" in this case are adjectives, and grammatically speaking saying the lamp is 2 feet tall and 15 pounds also describes the same object. However, are these descriptions the same? If no one is around to call it a lamp, it is still fundamentally a lamp, no matter the language or lack of language.

However, can this lamp be a "plain" or a "feng shui" lamp with no one to assess it as such? No actually, anything qualitative that could be said about the lamp remains with the people that own and use it. Linguistically though, qualitative and quantitative description/evaluation are communicated the same. Without this distinction with how we communicate quantitative and qualitative information, the quality of being a "plain" lamp sounds just as intrinsic as being a "2 foot tall" lamp.

A third opinion pops in and finds this lamp to be "tacky", and second opinion takes this a bit personally since they find the lamp to be intrinsically "feng shui". In this situation, both opinions can't be simultaneously correct, much like one can't be less than 3 feet tall and taller than 6 foot at the same time. On the other hand, if "tacky", "plain", or "feng shui" are just evaluations or judgments you're applying to the lamp rather than something that is the lamp itself, two or more contradicting evaluations can easily coexist. Having different opinions in itself does not create violence and chaos in the world, it is how we regard those differences in opinion that make or break this world.

It is all about individual perspective and taking into account where others are coming from and how that molds their perspective.

EXERCISE

1. I want you to pick one negative thought about yourself. If you can't think of any, let's just pick one of the following: "I know the NoPorn

plan will not work for me." Or "I'll never quit porn. I've tried it before. I've got not control over it."

There's no point in arguing whether a judgment or a story is true or not. What I'd like you to do is take a good look at what happens when you get caught up in one of your negative thoughts.

If you give this thought all your attention and let it dictate what you do, what happens to your life in the long run? Does getting caught up in this thought help you to be the person you want to be? Does it help you to do the things you want to do?

2. If your mind tells you for example that: "This won't work" and "you've got no control". That's normal. That's just the sort of stuff that minds say. I just want you to consider something; If we go along with that- if we let your mind dictate what happens- where do we go from here? Do we stop the program and give up?

I fully expect that your mind will continue telling you that you'll never quit porn. There's really no way to stop that from happening. So could we just allow our minds to tell us whatever they want, and just go on with this program anyway?

3. Whenever your mind says, "It's true I'm fat/stupid/ugly/a loser". Ask yourself: "When my mind says this to me, does it help me if I get all caught up in it or hold on to it? Does buying into these thoughts- giving them all my attention, allowing them to dictate what I do - does that help me in any way?

Write the answers to these questions in your journal.

MINDFULNESS EXERCISE

Ask a friend to read it to you alternatively you can get a recorded version of this exercise at nopornplan.com You will also get a comic book about porn addiction for free.

HANDS AS THOUGHTS

This exercise aims to explain the concept of Cognitive Defusion to you. There's no need to do this exercise repeatedly. Its purpose is just to illustrate a point.

Take a seat and imagine for a moment that your hands are your thoughts and rest them on your lap, palms up and open. Gradually raise your hands up toward your face until they've covered your eyes.

Now take a few seconds to look at the world around you through the gaps between your fingers. Notice how this interferes with your view.

I'd like you now to take a moment to think: What would it be like going through day-to-day activities with your hands covering your eyes like this? Take a while to think about this.

How much would it limit you? Take a while to think about this.

Could you effectively interact with the people around you like this? Take a while to think about this.

Would you be able to be to carry on with work or family matters like this? Take a while to think about this.

This is like fusion: We focus so much of our energy and attention on our thoughts that we disconnect from many aspects of our here-and-now experience. Our thoughts have such a significant impact over what we do, that our ability to act effectively in the present moment is substantially reduced.

Pause

Now start to lower your hands from your face very slowly.

Pause

As your hands slowly drop back onto your lap, notice how much easier it is to connect with your surroundings.

Pause

This is like defusion. like your hands, your thoughts don't disappear, but distancing them from you allows you to become more engaged with your life, allowing you to choose to act in ways that are aligned with your values instead of giving into your impulses. This is the end of this exercise.

LET'S PRACTICE COGNITIVE DEFUSION

Our minds are not our friends when we try to quit porn addiction. There's a part of our mind that actively tries to make us slip back into pornography. I personally have had a lot of experience with this. Whenever I got clean, my mind would eventually start talking to me and say things like "oh there's nothing wrong with looking at pictures" "Porn will not hurt you. Just allow yourself to use it for "a bit" or "You're so stressed. You need to unwind by using porn", then I would inevitably use porn again, and only after I had ejaculated all over my hands I realized what I'd done.

Minds also fuel our addiction in another way. Most porn addicts find that their porn addiction is fueled by negative self-evaluations and judgments. These act as major triggers for most people. Our minds not only very often try to persuade us to do porn, they also re-trigger us with negative self-evaluations such as "I'm a looser" or "I'm a failure."

We'll practice Cognitive Defusion a bit more which will help you to deal with coercion from your addicted self to do porn.

First I want you to understand that it's normal that your mind causes you trouble. In fact many psychologists will agree that this is what minds were designed to do. Minds have evolved millions of years ago. They have evolved for survival. Back in the Stone Age, your mind had to constantly look for danger, anticipating anything that could harm you in any way, "Could there be a wolf in these bushes?" In the Stone Age if you weren't vigilant, you died, and you didn't spread your genes, and as such only the cavemen who have turned their minds into a 'don't get killed' machine have survived and shaped how our minds are now. They were never evolved to help you achieve success or help you lead a happier and more fulfilling life. Minds have evolved to be critical, negative and judgmental because when you're afraid of everything and hate everything, you would most likely survive in the wilderness.

It wasn't a pleasant or successful life, but you lived, and that's all that evolution really cared about. That's why your mind always points out everything that could possibly go wrong. "You'll relapse", "There's no point in this", "you'll just fail again." This is just how minds were designed to function.

In a way, the mind is like a word machine that manufactures a never-ending stream of words. A radio of doom and gloom that likes to broadcast a lot of gloom about the past, and a lot of doom about the future, and a lot of dissatisfaction with the present.

It's also a spoiled brat. It makes all sorts of demands and throws a tantrum if it doesn't get its way. It's also a reason-giving machine: it churns out a never-ending list of reasons why you can't or shouldn't change.

That's just how minds were created. They were created for pure survival. Not for success, happiness, fulfillment or achievement.

Most people are slaves to these minds because they don't realize that there's another way. That's why in this lesson we'll learn how to turn your mind from your slave-owner into what it was meant to be, a tool you for you to use to improve your life. We'll achieve this by training you in one of the most powerful skills: Cognitive Defusion.

LET ME FURTHER ILLUMINATE TO YOU WHAT I MEAN BY COGNITIVE DEFUSION

Cognitive Defusion is difficult to grasp for many people. That's why I want to further illuminate the explanation I gave you in the previous lesson.

You can have two stances towards the content of your mind: You're either fused with it or you're defused from it. Fusion means you're getting caught up in your thoughts and allow them to control your behavior. In fusion you treat your thoughts as if they're you.

In defusion, you're separated and distanced from your thoughts, you let them come and go instead of being caught up in them. Defusion means looking at thoughts rather than from thoughts; noticing thoughts rather than being caught up in thoughts; and letting thoughts come and go rather than holding onto them.

In defusion, you see the true nature of thoughts. That they are nothing more but words, pictures, and sensations, and once you see their true nature, their power over you will diminish.

LET US LOOK AT THE DIFFERENT WAYS HOW FUSION MANIFESTS:

- Flashbacks
- Ruminating
- Worrying
- Trying to 'figure things out'
- Trying to 'figure my problems out'
- Trying to 'figure out how I'm like this'
- Trying to 'figure out why I'm like this'

Let me further illustrate this concept through metaphor:

You can be the driver in a bus, whilst all the passengers (thoughts) are being critical, abusive, intrusive, distracting, and shouting instructions, and sometimes even pure nonsense. You can allow the passengers to do as much noise as they want but all while keeping your attention at the road in front of you, heading towards your goal or value.

EXERCISES

REPEATING LEMON

This exercise involves three steps:

1. Pick a simple noun, such as "lemon." Say it out loud once or twice, and notice what it shows psychologically - what thoughts, images, smells, tastes, or memories come to mind? Now repeat the word over and over out loud as fast as possible for thirty seconds- until it becomes just a meaningless sound. Please try this now with the word "lemon," before you continue reading. You must do it out loud for it to be effective.

Now run through the exercise again with an evocative judgmental word - a word that you tend to use when you judge yourself harshly, for example, "bad," "fat," "idiot," "selfish," "loser," "incompetent,"--or a two-word phrase such as "bad mother." Please try this now and notice what happens. Most people find the word or phrase becomes meaningless within about thirty seconds. Then we see it for what it truly is: an odd sound, a vibration, a movement of mouth and tongue. But when that very same word pops into our head and we fuse with it, it has a lot of impact on us. Please try this exercise with any negative self-judgments and write about your experiences:

2. Have you listened to the hands as thought exercise?

Did it allow you to notice how your thoughts can disengage from the world? Try to write how you can relate this metaphor to your own experience with your thoughts, judgments and evaluations.

I'M HAVING THE THOUGHT THAT

To begin this exercise, first bring to mind an upsetting thought that takes the form "I am X." For example, "I'm not good enough" or "I'm incompetent." Preferably pick a thought that often recurs and that usually bothers or upsets you. Now focus on that thought and believe it as much as you can for ten seconds.

Next, take that thought and in front of it, insert this phrase: "I'm having the thought that ..." Play that thought again, but this time with the phrase attached. Think to yourself, "I'm having the thought that I am..." Notice what happens.

Now do that again, but this time the phrase is slightly longer: "I notice I'm having the thought that ..." Think to yourself, "I notice I'm having the thought that I am..." Notice what happens.

Did you do it? Remember, you can't learn to ride a bike just by reading about it; you actually have to get on the bike and pedal. And you won't get much out of this book if you just read the exercises. To change the way you handle your painful thoughts, you actually have to practice some new skills. So if you haven't done the exercise, please go back and do it now.

So what happened? You probably found that inserting those phrases instantly gave you some distance from the actual thought; as if you "stepped back" from it. (If you didn't notice any difference, try it again with another thought.)

You can use this technique with any unpleasant thought. For instance, if your mind says, "Life sucks!" then simply acknowledge, "I'm having the thought that life sucks!" If your mind says, 'I will fail!"

then simply acknowledge, "I'm having the thought that I'll fail!" Using this phrase means you're less likely to get beaten up or pushed around by your thoughts. Instead, you can step back and see those thoughts for what they are: nothing more than words passing through your head. We call this process "Defusion." In a state of fusion thoughts seem to be the absolute truth and very important. But in a state of defusion, we recognize that:

• Thoughts are merely sounds, words, stories, or bits of language.

• Thoughts may or may not be true; we don't automatically believe them.

• Thoughts may or may not be important; we pay attention only if they're helpful.

• Thoughts are definitely not orders; we certainly don't have to obey them.

• Thoughts may or may not be wise; we don't automatically follow their advice.

• Thoughts are never threats; even the most painful or disturbing of thoughts does not represent a threat to us.

In ACT we have many different techniques to facilitate defusion. Some of them may seem a bit gimmicky at first, but think of them like training wheels on a bicycle: once you can ride the bike, you don't need them anymore. So try out each technique as we come to it and see which works best for you. Remember as you use the techniques, the aim of defusion is not to get rid of a thought, but simply to see it for what it is -Just a string of words- and to let it be there without fighting it. Please do this exercise and write about your experience with it

MUSICAL THOUGHTS

Bring to mind a negative self-judgment that commonly bothers you when it comes up. For example, "I'm such an idiot." Now hold that thought in your mind and really believe it as much as you can for about ten seconds. Notice how it affects you.

Now imagine taking that same thought and singing it to yourself to the tune of "Happy Birthday." Sing it silently inside your head. Notice what happens.

Now go back to the thought in its original form. Once again, hold it in your mind and believe it as much as you can, for about ten seconds. Notice how it affects you. Write about your experiences

1. **Not Taking a Thought Seriously:** Bring to mind a thought that normally upsets you, that takes the form "I am X" (for example, "I am inadequate"). Hold that thought in your mind and notice how it affects you.

2. **Try Getting Intentionally Hooked:** Put your negative self-judgment into a short sentence--in the form, "I am x." For example, "I'm a loser" or "I'm not smart enough". Now fuse with this thought for ten seconds. In other words, get all caught up in it and believe it as much as you possibly can.

Now silently replay the thought with this phrase in front of it: "I'm having the thought that ..." For example, "I'm having the thought that I'm a loser." Now replay it one more time, but this time add this phrase "I notice I'm having the thought that ..." For example, "I notice I'm having the thought that I'm a loser."

What happened? Did you notice a sense of separation or distance from the thought? If not, run through the exercise again with a different thought. This is a nice simple exercise that gives an experience of defusion to almost everyone.

Did you get some sense of separation or distance from it? Write about your experience.

THE HAPPY BIRTHDAY TECHNIQUE:

Put your negative self-judgment into a short sentence -In the form "I am x"- and fuse with it for ten seconds.

Now, inside your head silently sing the thought to the tune "Happy Birthday."

Now, inside your head, hear it in the voice of a cartoon character, an actor, or a sport's commentator of your preference.

What happened that time? Did you notice a sense of separation or distance from the thought?

If not, run through the exercise again with a different thought.

Variations on the theme include singing the thoughts out loud, saying them out loud in a silly voice, or saying them in exaggerated slow motion. Write about your experience.

Now let's go through a specific defusion exercise called the Television screen. It will allow you to defuse unwanted visual thoughts with ease. Again either find a friend to read it to you or get the recorded version of this meditation at http://nopornplan.com

TELEVISION SCREEN

Think of an unpleasant image and notice how it's affecting you. Now imagine there's a small television in front of you. Place your image on the television screen. Play around with the image settings:

- **Flip it upside down.**
- **Turn it on its side.**
- **Spin it around.**
- **Play it in slow motion.**
- **Play it backwards.**
- **Play it forward in double speed.**
- **Turn the color down so it's all black and white.**
- **The idea is not to get rid of this image, but it see it for what it I; a harmless image. Nothing more.**

You may need to do it for a minute or two until you really defuse it

Pause
If you have trouble defusing from the unpleasant image, you might print over it with a funny line you've heard from a show or character, or try voicing it in your mind with a funny voice.
Pause
If you're still bothered by the image you might try to add a musical soundtrack of your choice to it. Try various kinds of music, including genres you like and dislike.
Pause
If the image is still bothering you, try imagining the image in a variety of different locations. Stay with each scenario for about twenty seconds before shifting to a new one. For example, visualize your image printed on a baseball cap.
Pause
Next as a commercial.
Pause
Then as a T-shirt design.
Pause
Then a billboard.

Pause

Try to visualize it as anything else that you can come up with. Use your imagination with this. The sky is the limit.

If you're still bothered by it, you might try some of the other defusion techniques you're learning in this book. At the end of the day everyone will have their own preferred technique. For example you can try the silly voices technique. Again either have a friend read it to you or get the recorded version at http://nopornplan.com

THE SILLY VOICES TECHNIQUE

While the television screen technique is highly visual, this defusion technique is highly auditory. Some people are more visual while some people are more auditory. I suggest you try both and see which technique you prefer. Of course, nothing stops you from using both. Find a thought that upsets you and focus on it for about ten seconds, believing in it as much as possible.

Pause

Notice how it affects you.

Now pick an animated cartoon character with a humorous voice, such as Peter Griffin, Daffy Duck, or Goofy. Now bring that troubling thought to mind but hear it in the cartoon character's voice, as if that character was speaking your thoughts out loud.

Pause

Notice what happens.

Pause

Now get the negative thought back in its original form and again try to believe it as much as possible. Notice what happens.

Pause

Now pick a different cartoon character with a funny voice. Gollum is a good choice. So is Yoda. Once again take that negative thought and hear it in that characters voice.

Notice what happens.

Pause

After repeating this a few times you will find that you're not taking the negative thought quite as seriously. You might even find yourself laughing at it.

Notice that you didn't change the thought or argue it away. You just saw it as what it is- a bit of language. By taking that segment of language and hearing it in a funny voice you become aware of its true nature. You become aware that it is nothing but a string of words, and because of that you defuse from it and it the thought loses its impact. Try practicing this technique each time you experience a particularly annoying thought that you can't get rid of.

[8]

How to Practice Mindfulness Even When You Struggle to Concentrate Because of Porn

SO FAR IN THIS PROGRAM we've discussed Cognitive Defusion and Willingness. Right now I want you to discuss another component of mindfulness, present moment awareness. Most popular meditation and mindfulness programs essentially equate mindfulness with present moment awareness, and as such I'll illuminate some of the most common definitions of mindfulness.

DEFINING MINDFULNESS AND PRESENT MOMENT AWARENESS

Most definitions of mindfulness emphasize present moment awareness. It could be helpful for you to learn them so you'll know exactly what skill you're training when you're practicing you're daily meditation practice with breathing meditation, the body scan, and other meditations in the noporn plan.

One of the most popular mindfulness authors, Jon Kabat Zin, defines mindfulness as:

"Paying attention in a particular way: on purpose, in the present moment, and nonjudgmentally"

Another textbook definition of mindfulness is:
"An open and receptive attention to and awareness of what is occurring in the present moment"

Yet another is:
"An awareness that arises through intentionally attending in an open, accepting and discerning way to whatever is arising in the present moment"

And the definition most commonly held by most Buddhist teachers is:
"Mindfulness is the unconditional awareness and acceptance of everything that happens in your present moment awareness."

WE KNOW THINGS BY KNOWING WHAT THEY'RE NOT: UNDERSTANDING MINDLESSNESS TO UNDERSTAND MINDFULNESS

Mindlessness occurs when attention and awareness scatter due to preoccupation with past memories or future plans and worries. This in turn leads to a limited awareness and attention to experiences in the present moment. So whenever you escape the present moment awareness into your thoughts of either the past or the future, you're being mindless and not mindful.

For most of my life I tried to be mindless. I can honestly mention at this point that for most of my life I actively did everything I could to be mindless. Being in the present moment forced me to tackle my negative emotions and my real life problems. In many ways I actively did everything I could do be mindless. I did porn, got involved in new age mysticism to escape my negative emotions, and spent most of my time practicing every other form of escapism I could get: video games, movies etc. All to escape my negative emotional experiences.

In **ACT**, this obstacle towards being mindful is called **Experiential Avoidance**, and it's something almost everyone has problems with. (Harris, 2009)

Being able to be with your negative emotions is a skill one has to develop FIRST to be in the present, this is why I've emphasized the Cognitive Defusion and acceptance before I tackled the subject of present moment awareness.

I remember the times when I tried to force myself to be present, without being able to present with my negative emotions. The result was always the same. I tried to observe my breath and do most of the meditations typically given by most meditation teachers, but sooner or later I would start being at war with myself. I would fight my emotions and the present moment experience.

MINDFULNESS IS NOT RELIGIOUS OR SPIRITUAL, IT'S PSYCHOLOGICAL

Mindfulness is a psychological skill that's unaligned with any religion. Practicing mindfulness does not make you a Buddhist, Hindu, Christian, Muslim or religious in any way. If you don't want to be, you don't even have to be spiritual.

Although practicing mindfulness by having a regular meditation practice will make you a better Buddhist, Christian, Hindu or Muslim if you persistently do it every day.

Although relaxation helps with being mindful. Relaxation is not the goal of being mindful. Mindfulness is not relaxation. Relaxation is not mindfulness.

You might have noticed that we often include a progressive relaxation before certain meditation techniques. We do it because we find that being relaxed makes mindfulness easier. But we want to emphasize that relaxation is not the goal of mindfulness. The goal of mindfulness is to allow you to be present with your experience no matter whether it's pleasant or unpleasant. It's just that it's easier to train that skill when you're relaxed. That's why we have a progressive relaxation in the beginning of many of our meditations.

Meditation is generally much harder for westerners than for people in the east. It's especially hard for us porn addicts since once we progress to harder fetish porn each time we masturbate to porn, we fill our subconscious mind with disturbing images which make our minds far more prone to resist the present moment.

To really explain this effect porn has on our ability to be present, I want to refer to ancient energetic explanations of our bodies.

In ancient times people explained their psyche using metaphors. The most popular metaphor for the psyche was the energy system composed of chakras, meridians and other esoteric components. Practitioners of Chinese medicine and Ayurveda have hypothesized that regular porn use disrupts this energetic system, making it harder for our mind to become focused and steady in meditation. (Sivananda, 1960)

An alternative explanation comes from the field of Psychodynamic psychotherapy, specifically body-based psychotherapy. Wilhelm Reich has postulated a sexual energy in our bodies called Orgone, which is directly disturbed by porn use. (Reich, 1973) His successor Alexander Lowen also postulated a similar type of energy which he called 'bioenergetics'. (Willis, 2010)

The difference between the energies postulated by ancient mystics and the energies in psychodynamic psychotherapy practiced in the 21st century is that modern psychotherapists treat these energies more like an metaphor for subjective experience of physiological changes in our bodies and brains that happen as a result of trauma and extensive porn use. Specifically Wilhelm Reich and Alexander

Lowen have linked it to the creation of chronic muscle tensions in our bodies that essentially store our past traumas. They referred to this as 'body armoring'. (Lowen, 1994).

HOW PORN HURTS YOU ACCORDING TO BIOENERGETIC THEORY

As you know by now, porn addiction progresses in such a way that we masturbate to harder and harder stuff. I first started masturbating to softcore porn, and then progressed to torture porn. Each time I went to more depraved porn, it this left a very profound mark on my psyche, making it harder for me to meditate or to even focus on basis daily tasks. I know that many of you might experience a similar difficulty with meditating. That's why I want you to give you a meditation that's been practiced for millennia, designed specifically for people whose psyche has been contaminated by trauma, porn or other more serious mental turmoil.

If you don't agree with the esoteric or psychodynamic explanation, don't worry this meditation will still be helpful to you

There's a very simple alternative explanation as to why this meditation helps people train mindfulness skills even when they find it difficult to sit through sitting meditations such as the body-scan meditation or the breathing meditation. This meditation is simply far more stimulating than regular meditation, and as such someone who has problems or is simply unaccustomed to sitting still for extended periods of time will find it easier to attend to this meditation.

EXERCISE: WILLINGNESS WITH AN AVATAR

The alternative to trying to control, change, fix, magnify, or minimize a thought or feeling is willingness. Willingness can be described in a number of ways: as allowing our thoughts and feelings to be as they are, regardless of whether they are pleasant or painful; as opening up and making room for our thoughts and feelings; as dropping the struggle with them; as letting them come and go as they naturally do; or simply as showing up for the present moment.

This can be a little abstract, so I'd like to ask you to do an exercise that can make it more concrete. One useful way to get a sense of what willingness is like is to represent your thought or feeling in an object and act willingly with that object. It sounds a little weird, but it can be very helpful. Here's what I'm going to ask you to do: I'd like you to come up with an object to represent a difficult feeling or thought you have. It can be a ball, a rock, a stuffed animal, an index card - Anything you have available with you. (A small stuffed animal can be useful because it's hard to fight or suppress something that's cute).

Over the next week, treat this object -And the thought or feeling- like it's something welcome that doesn't need to go away. Here are some ways you can do that: You can carry it around with you and keep it nearby when you're working, studying, eating meals, dedicating yourself to your hobbies and anywhere you go. It can be in your bag, on a table next to you, or in your hand. Occasionally, interact with it in a way that's welcoming and caring. For example, hold it gently like something precious, or keep it next to you while you're working on your computer, like it's your sidekick. If it's a stuffed animal, pet it. Throughout the week, mindfully notice any urges to reassure, fix, or change your object. From time to time, hold it in your hand and notice that it's distinct from you and not the whole of you, just like your difficult feeling or thought. Notice that your awareness of it comes and goes, just like your feeling or thought. Notice that you can let it just be there, or you can focus on it very intently, just like your feeling or thought.

Treat it like an invited guest. You might even say something like "Come on in, sadness, and have a seat." Remember, you don't have to like it to welcome it.

Wherever you keep it, give it space to be. Keep in mind that being present is neither goal oriented nor intended to achieve an outcome. It's simply being with whatever shows up in the moment. There's nothing fancy here. All we're doing is trying to practice interacting with thoughts and feelings in a different way. Notice that we aren't trying to change your thoughts and feelings; rather, we're trying to change your relationship with your thoughts and feelings. We're building a skill that will allow you to experience a feeling in the moment and also do what's important to you at the same time.

CATHARTIC MEDITATION: MEDITATION FOR PEOPLE WHO FIND IT HARD TO MEDITATE

The cathartic meditation is based on practice done by mystics such as sufis, druids, spinning dervishes and tribal shamans for decades. A version of this meditation has been popularized by the popular spiritual mystic Osho: an eastern spiritual master who worked with westerners. He has noticed that some of his disciples have done a form of this meditation spontaneously. He then modified it and sold it using the name "dynamic meditation". The difference between Cathartic Meditation and Dynamic Meditation is that Osho's dynamic meditation includes a few unnecessary steps such as freezing in place while standing, which make it less enjoyable and more difficult to practice on a regular basis. I've made this meditation far more enjoyable and adjusted it for daily practice.

The additional bonus of this cathartic meditation is that it's also a good cardio workout. As you'll learn in a lesson further in the program, physical exercise has been proven to be helpful in elevating all addictive urges, and doing this meditation for 20 minutes is essentially an equivalent to running for 20 minutes on an elliptical.

How to Do The Cathartic Meditation

You can get an instructional video explaining this meditation at http://nopornplan.com On that website you can also get a free comic book that will illustrate the things you're learning in this book.

Stage #1 (ten minutes): Start by standing with your eyes closed and breathe deep and fast through your nose continuously. If you are only physically capable of doing deep breathing for five minutes, then reduce the length of the first stage. Remember that you are doing this method to help your meditation, not to physically injure yourself. Allow your body to move freely as you breathe. You can jump up and down, sway back and forth, or use any physical motion that helps you pump more oxygen into your lungs.

Stage #2 (twenty minutes): The second stage is a celebration of catharsis and wild and spontaneous dancing. Totally let go and act as an ancient human dancing in tribal celebration. Energetic, nonverbal background music is recommended. African tribal drum music works especially well. You may roll on the ground and do strange spontaneous body movements. Allow your body to move within the limits so long you're not hurting yourself or others. Screaming is encouraged. You must act out any anger you may have in a safe way, such as beating the earth with your hands. All of the suppressed emotions from your subconscious mind are to be released. If at any time during the second stage you feel that your energy level is starting to decline, you can resume deep and fast breathing to give yourself a boost.

Stage #3 (ten minutes): This stage is complete quiet and relaxation. Lay down on your back, get comfortable, and just let go. Just observe whatever happens in your body and your environment. Optimally you'd practice the open awareness mindfulness exercise at this stage. But any mindfulness exercise will do. From the energetic perspective regularly practicing the cathartic meditation will help release energetic blocks caused by porn. From a psychodynamic perspective it will help release stored traumas in the body. And from a more skeptical cognitive-behavioral perspective, this meditation is simply way easier to focus on and will allow you to practice being present even if you find observing your breath to be too hard at this point.

Note: Make sure you have enough space to practice this meditation, and wait at least 30 minutes after eating before doing it.

How To Startup a Mindfulness Practice

I know I've given you a lot to process during this module. That's why I want to give you a very short lesson this time. Today's lesson is all about how to startup a mindfulness practice.

I know that the high amount of mindfulness exercises I provided might seem overwhelming. But it's really less than it seems to be at first glance. Most of the exercises given to you here are designed to illustrate a therapeutic point or to teach you a technique you'll use when it's needed. For example the silly voices technique and the television screen technique audio recordings show you techniques you can use when you have a thought you want to get rid of. They are not meant to be practiced regularly.

Only a few of the exercises in this book are actually 'push-ups' for your mindfulness muscles

Allow me to list the exercises that designed for regular mindfulness practice:

- **Mindfulness of breathing**
- **Mindfulness of the body**
- **Mindfulness of emotions**
- **The conveyor belt exercise**
- **The cathartic meditation**

Now there is some of which you have not been yet introduced too. But you'll learn them soon:

- **The compassion exercises**
- **Open awareness exercise (which you'll learn in this chapter)**

After you read these lessons a few times you'll be able to do them on your own. Alternatively if you get a friend to read them to you you'll also be able to learn them well enough to practice them on your own. And doing them shouldn't take you more than 10 minutes. Most of them initially take longer because you're learning them. But once you learn them you it's actually very easy to use them daily.

Here are some tips on creating a mindfulness practice:

Make it a habit by doing it every day at the same time of day: Practice at the same time every day to make it a habit. When we do a thing every time we wake up or just before going to bed we'll always remember to do it. When was the last time you forgot to brush your teeth? You probably didn't have that experience very often. Because it has become a habit. You created that habit by doing it every day at the same time of the day.

Be gentle with yourself: At the end of the day you really can't do mindfulness wrong. If you're practicing mindfulness. You're doing it correctly. Remember that

It's optimal for you to do mindfulness while sitting with your back straight: But remember that's just the optimum. If you practice mindfulness while slouching or lying down it will still work. The 'keep your back straight' thing is only there to keep you from falling asleep. (Ps. If you fall asleep while doing mindfulness try doing it with your back straight).

Remember 10 minutes per day is enough: Even 5 minutes per day is enough. Doing 5-10 minutes per day is better than doing an hour session per week.

Remember that you can practice mindfulness while doing other things: As I have taught you in previous lessons many daily activities allow us to practice mindfulness. During the course of the day you'll probably be forced to wash dishes, clean, or at the very least eat. Use any one of these activities to practice mindfulness, and you'll be able to practice mindfulness without wasting a second of your time, since you'll just be using an activity you have to do anyway.

Set a timer: This is not for everyone, but many people find that if they say to themselves "I'll practice mindfulness for 10 minutes per day" and then set a timer for 10 minutes before practicing mindfulness they'll find it easier to follow through.

You can even use it as a sleeping aid: Remember how I told you that keeping your back straight is made to keep you from falling asleep? Well it's because when you're laying down there is a real tendency for you to relax, which in turn might make you fall asleep. This won't happen immediately but probably 10 minutes in. And as such if you have trouble sleeping you can simply practice mindfulness until you fall asleep. The compassion exercise which you'll learn in the relationship section is especially good for this, so is the body awareness exercise.

But remember - The point of living is living, not meditating or doing therapy. While meditation can be pleasurable and it is useful. At the end of the day it is pretty much the mental equivalent of strength training: It is useful and can make you stronger, but I don't want you to make all your life about it. I'm not saying you shouldn't value mindfulness. But there is difference between exercising regularly and being a bodybuilder. You don't need to be a mental bodybuilder to recover from porn. You don't need to meditate 1 hour per day. 10 - 20 minutes per day is more than enough. Similarly someone who's overweight doesn't really need to exercise for 4 hours per day to lose weight.

Ultimately the way to overcome porn is the find what you want your life to be about and do it. That's why in the next session we'll help you figure out exactly what you want your life to be about.

OPEN AWARENESS MEDITATION

Again either have a friend read this meditation to you or get the recorded version at http://nopornplan.com

This exercise is considered to be the most difficult and most challenging of the mindfulness exercises in this course. It essentially distills the essence of mindfulness and asks you to practice it in a relatively unstructured environment. So just let go of expectations and demands on yourself and let yourself as you do this. Even though this mindfulness exercise might be challenging, you cannot really do this wrong. As long as you notice that you're distracted and return to the exercise, you're still training your mindfulness muscles.

Now sit with your back straight and close your eyes.

Pause

Now focus on your breathing. Just for a few seconds practice mindfulness of breathing. You already know how to practice it, without guidance.

Pause

Just observe the breath as if you've never seen it before, and whenever a thought comes up let it pass by like a car passing by in the street, and gently allow your attention to go back to your breath.

Now allow your breathing to find its natural rhythm. Let go of control and let your breathing to be as it is, while observing it with an attitude of openness, acceptance and curiosity

Now expand your awareness so that you're aware of other parts of your experience. Become aware of your body. The position of your body in your chair, your body posture.

Now expand your awareness again, and become aware of your thoughts. Notice your thoughts. Where do they appear? How do they manifest?

Now expand your attention a bit more so you become aware the sounds around you. Both the sounds outside of you and within in you

Now simply allow yourself to open up to the present moment as it is, and allow everything to be as it is. Just make it your intention to be fully open to the present moment and notice what's happening with an attitude of openness and interest.

Now. Simply practice awareness. There's no need for you to direct your attention in any way. Simply observe whatever shows up.

If thoughts catch your attention, observe your thoughts.

If breathing catches your attention, then observe your breath

If feelings catch your attention, observe your feelings

You may observe multiple aspects of your experience at the same time. For example you might be aware of your breathing at the same time as you're aware of the feelings in your body.

If at any point you fuse with your thoughts and become completely engulfed by your mind or if you just get distracted by anything else, simply return your attention to observing whatever arises.

Long Pause for 2 Minutes

Eventually, instead of observing your mind, you'll get caught up by it. You might become tangled up in feelings or lost in thoughts, which will make you lose your observer perspective.

When you've realized that this has happened, simply defuse yourself from your thoughts and once again take an observer perspective, observing whatever it was that carried you away.

Whatever you're observing. Simply allow it to be as it is. Don't cling to it, but also don't try to push it away. Just notice it and allow it to be there.

Whether it's a thought a sensation, a feeling or sound, just notice it, allow it to be there, and observe it.

Long Pause 2 Minute Pause

Take a moment to notice that there are the feelings, sensations, sounds, thoughts, and smells you're observing it, and that there's the "you" that's observing them. Realize that since you're observing them, you cannot be them.

Pause

If at any point you become lost and disoriented come back to your breath and follow it for a few seconds, and then once again practice observing whatever shows up in your present moment awareness.

Many people find remaining to be an observer challenging. Your thoughts and feelings will distract you from your observing self. That's normal. When you've noticed this, simply come back to observing whatever's arising in your awareness.

Pause

Whenever you get carried away by a thought or feeling, simply take a moment to let ig go, and go back to observing. Whenever you feel disoriented. Observe your breath for a few seconds, and then go back to observing whatever arises in your present moment awareness.

Pause

Now expand your awareness and notice everything that's happening in your present moment awareness. Notice your body, notice your breathing, notice the sounds in the room, and notice your feelings.

Open your eyes and notice what you can see. Expand your awareness so that you notice everything that's happening around you. Enter the present moment fully.

Congratulate yourself for finishing up this exercise, and that you've learned a technique to train your mindfulness muscles.

USING MINDFULNESS FOR EMOTIONAL MANAGEMENT WITH THE MINDFUL QUESTION METHOD

Most porn addicts find that they use porn to cope with negative emotions and with difficult life circumstances. That's why I decided to devote an entire lesson to the subject of emotional management. Most techniques that deal with this subject claim that they are teaching you some 'super-secret technique' that tries to get 'rid' of your emotions. There are techniques that can desensitize some very strong feelings of anxiety and depression and you'll actually learn all of these techniques later. However, the truth is that those techniques are not magic, they only essentially 'turn off' those very strong pathological feelings, and most of the time they just tone them down to manageable levels. The truth is that you'll always experience some levels of emotional discomfort from time to time, because that's just simply how humans are built. There's no such thing as happiness without a moment of unhappiness. Throughout history, there have been many charlatans who have claimed to sell enlightenment and positioned it as something akin to happiness without a moment unhappiness, but the truth is that everyone no matter what technique they use or what they know about human psychology, will experience some negative emotions from time to time. The only way for you to truly deal with them is for you to manage them. The truth is that from the perspective of quitting porn addiction and getting greater success in life, negative emotions (except the very strong negative emotions that you'll learn to manage through a technique called **TAAP** and acupressure desensitization which will be discussed in the future) are not by themselves problematic. In fact, they usually start as very mild experiences. We simply make them stronger by our judgments and our resistance to them.

When you struggle and try to 'get rid' of negative emotions:

• Your emotions become stuck.

• You waste a huge amount of time and energy on struggling with them.

• By fighting your emotions and struggling with them, you generate suffering.

On the other hand, when you don't struggle with emotions and simply open up to them, and allow them to be there without being controlled by them:

• Your emotions are free to move

• You don't waste time fighting your emotions or trying to avoid them

• You don't suffer

In essence there's a simple equation that explains the cause of all suffering:

Pain x Resistance = Suffering

If your resistance to your pain (physical or emotion) is "0" then your suffering is "0". It's as simple as that.

Now today's meditation will train this skill directly, but I also want to give you a very simple technique for emotional management I created called the **Mindful Question Method**. It's designed to prompt you to be present with your emotional experience by asking you a series of carefully crafted questions. Our minds tend to remember questions and words more than abstract concepts. Additionally, some psychologists speculate that questions are able to elicit a direct response from our unconscious mind.

If you find yourself facing an emotion that prompts a 'No' answer to any of these questions, I would like you to simply use a technique that I'll teach you later called **TAAP**, which is designed to deal with stronger, more overwhelming emotions. **TAAP** is more cumbersome to implement and it's not really designed to deal with every emotion you experience, and as such I would like you to become proficient with the mindful question method first, and then progress into **TAAP**.

The mindful question method is composed of 4 steps. Each composed of a series of questions:

Step 1: Become aware of your experience. Could I just be aware of this experience as it is? Just see whether or not you can become aware of this experience as it is. We're not trying to change it or control it in any way. Just see whether or not you can become aware of this experience as it is.

Could I just observe this experience like a curious scientist?

Just allow yourself to observe this experience like a curious scientist. Focus on the sensation you experience in that moment. Notice where it starts and where it stops. Notice its shape. Notice how it feels. Is it heavy or light? Is it pulsating or throbbing? Is it hot or cold?

Step 2: Ground yourself. Could I become aware of my breath and body?

Just become aware of your breathing. This acts as an anchor that keeps you centered in the emotional storm.

Step 3: Open Up and make space. Could I open up to this experience? Could I make space for this experience?

Just see if you could open up to this experience. Could you just make space for it? We're not trying to change or control it. Just see if you could open up to this experience. As if you're giving it space to move. Generally we constrict ourselves around negative emotional experience. We get stressed about our stress and anxious about anxiety. This fuels our negative experience. Instead I would like you to see whether or not you could open up to this experience. (If this experience is too strong, don't worry. We have another technique to deal with emotions like that. For now use it with emotions that are not too overwhelming or strong).

Step 4: Allow. Could I allow this experience to just be there as it is, even if I don't like it or want it? Could I just let it be?
Now see if you could allow this experience to be exactly as it is. Just for now. Could you just be with it? Just see if you if you could allow it to be there without judgment. When you notice your mind commenting on what's happening just say "Thanks mind" and come back to observing your present moment experience. At first this will be difficult you'll feel a strong urge to fight this urge or push it away. That's normal. If you notice it acknowledge that urge as if you nodded in recognition and said "There you are; I see you". Then bring your attention right back to the sensation.
Remember. The goal of this technique is not to get rid of this sensation or alter it, just to take back its control over you. Sometimes it might change by itself, but that's unintentional. If it happens that's okay, if not that's okay too. The goal is for you to let the emotion be there even if you don't want it or like it. You might need to focus on this emotion for a while for you to give up struggling with it. That's okay. Learning a valuable skill like this takes time.
Once you've done this see if there's some other troublesome sensation and repeat the procedure. Keep doing this until you completely stop struggling with your current present moment experience.

Optional: If you notice yourself get fused with a particularly strong thought you can ask yourself "Could I defuse from this thought?" This will allow you to move back to the present moment, experience and focus on it.

Once you'll become proficient at this technique your feelings will have far less impact on you. You'll still feel them or you might not. That doesn't matter. What matters is that they won't have any emotional control over you. That they won't trigger your porn addiction and make you relapse on porn. That's all that matters.

And after you become more proficient with this technique all you'll need to do is ask yourself "Could I open up to this experience?" And focus on your breathing, and then ask "Could I defuse from this thought?" Each time you're distracted by a thought. This whole procedure will take seconds with practice.

For today's homework I would like to pick 3 negative memories or negative emotions. I want you to pick something relatively mild. Not a major phobia or anything like that. Just a regular stress or something that you find irritating. It's important for you to pick something mild at first. Such as being annoyed by your neighbor.

Labeling can also help you defuse emotions.

You can also defuse emotions by labeling them. Which you'll learn in this guided meditation called Mindfulness of Emotions and either have someone read it to you or get the recorded version at http://nopornplan.com

In this exercise you'll learn a very powerful technique for managing your emotions. Before we start it I'd like you to pick up a small object, anything will do. Now I want you to grasp it as strongly as you can. Just squeeze it in your hand as tightly as you can. This is what we do with our emotions when we resist them. Now I want you to simply open up your palm, and see how the objects fall from your hand. This is what happens when we allow emotions to be as they are.

When we resist emotions we get stressed about our stress and angry about our anger, which in turn increases our stress and anger, for example.

Practicing mindfulness with your emotions allows you to let go of your struggle with them, which in the long run helps you to manage them better. In this mindfulness exercise we're simply aiming for you to let go of your resistance to your emotions, to let go of fighting them. Our aim is not to make you like them or love them or make them 'go away'. We're making room for them and allowing them to be as they are even if we don't like them. Doing this will allow you to experience emotions without being controlled by them. By practicing this technique repeatedly you'll eventually learn how to feel your emotion without being behaviorally controlled by them. This way you won't have to repress or hide your emotions, but you also won't have to be a slave to them.

To reiterate: In this exercise we're allowing our emotions to be as they are. We'll be observing them like a curious scientist might observe a butterfly.

So sit down with your back straight and close your eyes.

Pause

Now for a few seconds, focus on your breathing.

Pause

Now bring to mind a situation that brings up bad feelings in you. Don't choose anything too traumatic. Just something that's essentially an average bad thing that might happen to you. For a few minutes allow yourself to think about this problem.

A good strategy for emotional management is to go into your body each time you feel a negative emotions. That's why as you're thinking about your problem, I'd like you to take a deep breath and scan your body from your toes to the top of your head.

Pause

As you do that notice what sensations this problem creates in your body. Does the emotions produce sensations in your stomach? Your head? Your chest? Or anywhere else?

Just scan your body and notice any strong sensations in your body that are associated with this unpleasant emotion you're experiencing right now.

If you notice several uncomfortable sensations, look for the strongest sensation. The one that's bothering you're the most. It might be heaviness in your stomach or tightness in your chest. Focus all of your attention on that sensation and observe it with curiosity and acceptance, as if you're a friendly scientist observing a butterfly or any other wild animal.

As a friendly scientist you're not trying to get rid or destroy the creature you're observing. You're simply studying it, allowing it to be there. Allow yourself to observe this sensation, notice where it starts and where it ends, learning as much about it as you can.

- If you could draw a line around his sensation, what would it look like?
- Is it on the surface of your body or on the inside?
- Where is the sensation the strongest?
- Where is it weakest?
- Does it pulsate?
- Does it vibrate?
- Is it moving?
- What is its weight; is it heavy or light?
- What is its perceived temperature?

Allow yourself to observe the sensation with an attitude of interest and openness.

Now take a deep breath and allow yourself to let go of all your resistance to this sensation. You don't have to like it or want it, or approve of it. Simply let go of your resistance to it, and allow it to be as
it is.

Just make room for it. Just allow it to be there as it is. If you feel any
resistance to it building up, simply allow yourself to allow the resistance to be there, and observe it as a curious scientist might observe a lion eating a zebra

You don't have to like it. But simply make room for it, and allow it to
be there.

Just allow yourself to observe the sensations. Don't think about the
sensations, when your mind starts commenting no what's happening, simply let these thoughts come and go, and gently redirect your
attention to the sensations that you're observing.

Your mind will repeatedly take your attention away from these sensations, and every time it happens just allow these thoughts to come
and go, like cars passing by, and move your attention back to observing the emotional sensations you're experiencing right now.

Pause

Whenever you find that you get caught up by the thoughts. Just notice what happened and return to observing

Pause

Again observe the emotional sensation. Notice its size and shape. Allow it to be there. Make room for it.

Pause

You don't have to like it or want it, just allow the sensation to be
there. Notice the difference between how your mind tells you the
sensation is, and how the sensation actually is.

Your mind might tell you that the sensation is too painful or too overwhelming, but when it does, just let these thoughts pass by like cars
passing by, and return your attention to the sensation.

You might find doing this exercise difficult. Your mind might create a strong urge to fight with this sensation, to make it go away, to push it away, to repress it. If that happens simply acknowledge this urge without giving into it, and gently bring your attention back to the emotional sensation you are observing. Notice its texture, notice its weight, notice how it feels. You might notice that this particular sensation is made up of smaller sensations, which subsequently are made up of even smaller sensation.

Don't try to get rid of the sensation. Don not try to change it. If it changes by itself that okay, but if it doesn't that's okay too. All you need to do is to observe it; to allow it to be there as it is, without trying to change it.

In mindfulness we don't aim to change the feeling, we simply want you to allow it to be as it is, to let go of your resistance to it, and notice it with an attitude of openness and interest.

Simply notice the sensation, and allow it to be there. Do it for a few minutes.

Pause For a Minute

Notice the sensation and allow it be there.

Pause For 30 Seconds

Notice the sensation and allow it be there.

Pause For 30 Seconds

Notice the sensation and allow it be there.

Pause For 30 Seconds

Notice the sensation and allow it be there.

Pause For 30 Seconds

Notice the sensation and allow it be there.

Pause For 30 Seconds

During this exercise your mind will create judgments and thoughts that will distract you from the sensation in your body, the moment you realize that you're distracted, simply gently return to observing these sensations. Make room for them and allow them to be there exactly as they are

Pause For 30 Seconds
Notice the sensation and allow it be there.
Pause For 30 Seconds
Notice the sensation and allow it be there.
Pause For 30 Seconds
Notice the sensation and allow it be there.
Pause For 30 Seconds

Once you feel that you've let go of all your resistance to this sensation, simply scan your body again and see if there's another uncomfortable sensation created by the unpleasant emotional experience you were thinking about, and if there is one, simply repeat this procedure with the new sensation. Just observe it with curiosity and openness like a friendly scientist would observe an interesting finding.

- What is its shape?
- What is its texture?
- Observe its weight
- Observe its temperature
- Simply allow it to be as it is

Each time you're distracted by your thoughts or taken away by your thoughts or fused with your thoughts, simply notice it and come back to observing this emotional sensation with an attitude of curiosity and openness.
Pause
If a thought distracts you, just let it pass as you would a group of birds in the sky.
Pause

Just notice as much of the sensation as you can. Observe it, without thinking about it. Your mind will create thoughts, but let these ideas and thoughts come and go, while observing this sensation with openness, interest and curiosity, even if you don't like it. Like you would watch a sad or scary movie on television.

Pause

Now as we're coming to the end of this exercise, let everything go and return to your breathing. Observe your breath for a few seconds.

Pause

Allow your attention to expand, become aware of the feeling of your body, of the sound of my voice, and your breathing simultaneously. Allow yourself to become aware of your entire environment.

And open your eyes and congratulate yourself on doing this exercise.

Try to do this each time you feel a negative emotion. This will help you better manage them. It will allow you to observe them like you are observing something on television, which will allow you to be aware of your emotions without being controlled by your emotions. Additionally repeatedly doing this exercise will train your mindfulness skills, which in turn will allow you to do the same thing you're doing with emotions regarding your urges for porn and other things you wouldn't like you to do.

In an technique you'll see a future lesson you'll learn how to do what you're doing with emotions now with your addictive urges, which will allow you be aware of them, without being controlled by them. But for now try to regularly practice this technique.

[9]

FEAR and How It Causes Your Porn Addiction.

I WANT YOU TO UNDERStand that you're not your addiction and that your addicted thoughts don't define you. I want to give you a few metaphors that illustrate this point.

YOUR TRUE SELF IS LIKE THE SKY

Thoughts and feelings are like the weather. The weather changes constantly, but no matter how bad it gets, it cannot harm the sky in any way. The mightiest thunderstorm, the most turbulent hurricane, the most severe winter blizzard -These things cannot harm the sky. No matter how bad the weather, the sky always has room for it- and sooner or later, the weather always clears up. Now sometimes we forget the sky is there, but it never changes its place. Sometimes we can't see the sky -It's obscured by clouds. But if we rise high enough, above those clouds- even through the thickest, darkest, thunderclouds -we'll eventually reach clear sky, stretching in all directions, boundless and pure.

IT'S ALSO LIKE A CHESSBOARD

As you keep practicing, you can learn to access this part of you: a safe space inside of you from which to observe and make room for difficult thoughts and feelings. Imagine a chessboard, where the white pieces are all your positive thoughts and feelings, and the black pieces are all your negative ones. We go through life desperately trying to move our white pieces across and wipe off all the black pieces. But the problem is; there are an infinite number of white and black pieces. No matter how many black pieces you wipe off, more will appear. Also, black pieces will attack white pieces. You move forward the white piece, "I'm a good parent," and immediately the black piece attacks, "No, you're not. What about the time yelled at your kids?" So we can go through life, wasting a lot of time and energy, trying to win this battle that can never be won and never ends. Or we can learn how to be more like the chessboard. The board is in intimate contact with all the pieces, but it's not involved in the battle. There's a part of us that operates like this chessboard. In ACT, we call it the observing self. It enables us to step out of the battle with our thoughts and feelings while giving them plenty of space to move around.

IN A WAY YOU'RE LIKE A CLASSROOM

Your thoughts and feelings are like the students in the classroom: Some are negative, some are positive, and some are neutral. There's also a part of you that tends to evaluate your thoughts and feelings. Like the teacher, it probably tries to make the negative thoughts pipe down and attempts to keep the positive thoughts around by giving them a gold star. But there is another part to this metaphor: the classroom that contains the students and the teacher. It's in close contact with them yet also separate from them. It's the context that contains them. So perhaps you aren't the students or the teacher--the thoughts, feelings, or evaluations -But the classroom- the vessel that simply contains those experiences. Your true self doesn't change.

This metaphor might illustrate what I mean by this: Doesn't it seem as though your early life was such a battle that you had to put on strong armor to defend yourself? You became a knight, constantly at war and therefore keeping your armor on all the time. You got so comfortable in your armor that it was like an extension of your own body and you forgot you were wearing it. And it worked. It stopped you from being hurt. Look at your life now. Are you still in a battle with people around you? Could it be that the war is over, but you're still clunking around inside this suit of armor? How free are you to move? What is the armor really costing you?

While it's true that wearing the armor keeps you from being hurt is it also stopping you from having the feeling from being held, being loved? What would it feel like to take off armor that seems to no longer fit?

The self-as concept is hard to understand the English language because it doesn't have a word to properly describe it. Let's look at how other cultures describe this: In the Kikongo language, spoken in the Democratic Republic of Congo, the word for "people" is "Bantu". The singular form of this word is "Muntu". Muntu, unlike the English "Person," refers not only to a living person, but beings that have yet to be born, as well as those who have died. Muntu is a transcendent self that persists, stably and unchanged, through prelife, life, and afterlife. The Congolese speak of Muntu as a Self that exists inside the body but separate from it, looking out through the eyes and simply watching what occurs. This self doesn't get attached to outcomes because it isn't affected by them and it can't die. It's a self that simply transitions from spirit to body and back again.

This is much like the ACT concept of self-as context: A stable, unchanging self that transcends the content of thoughts and feelings - A self that experiences and contains these elements but isn't defined by them.

NOW LET ME EXPLAIN A FEW PSYCHOLOGICAL DEFINITIONS THAT ARE ILLUSTRATED IN THESE METAPHORS

SELF-CONCEPT: This is the story you have about yourself. In this state you think that you're your thoughts, you're fused with them.

SELF-AS AWARENESS: This is the ongoing process of noticing experience, and contacting the present moment.

SELF-AS-CONTEXT: This is the space from which noticing happens. When you have observed your breath in the last exercises who did the noticing? Who notices these words as you read them? This is the self-as context. Pure awareness.

Now we'll do an exercise that will let you experience your 'self-as context' either have a friend read it to you or get the recorded at http://nopornplan.com

Sit down in a comfortable position and start breathing. Notice the breath flowing in and out of your lungs. Notice it coming in through the nostrils. Down into the lungs. And back out again. And as you do that, be aware you're noticing where your breath goes, and there you are noticing it.

Pause For 5 Seconds

If you can notice your breath, you cannot be your breath.

Pause For 5 Seconds

Your breath changes continually, sometimes shallow, sometimes deep, sometimes fast, sometimes slow, but the part of you that notices your breath does not change.

Pause For 5 Seconds

And when you were a child, your lungs were so much smaller, but then the only person that could notice your breathing as a child is the same you have become now.

Now that gets your mind whirring, analyzing, philosophizing, and debating. So take a step back and notice, where are your thoughts? Where are they located? Are they moving or still? Are they pictures or words?

Pause For 5 Seconds

And as you do notice your thoughts, be aware you're taking notice, there go your thoughts, and there you are noticing them.

Pause For 5 Seconds

If you can notice your thoughts, you cannot be your thoughts.

Pause For 5 Seconds

Your thoughts change continually, sometimes true, sometimes false, sometimes positive, sometimes negative. Sometimes happy and sometimes sad. But the part of you that notices your thoughts does not change.

Pause For 5 Seconds

And when you were a child, your thoughts were so very different than they are today, but the you who could notice your thoughts as a child is the same you takes notice of them as an adult.

Pause For 5 Seconds

Now I don't expect your mind to agree to this. In fact, I expect throughout the rest of this exercise your mind will debate, analyze, or attack whatever I say, so see if you can let those thoughts come and go like passing cars, and engage in the exercise no matter how hard your mind tries to pull you away.

Pause For 5 Seconds

Now notice your body in the chair.

Pause For 5 Seconds

And as you do that, be aware you're noticing, there is your body, and there you are noticing it. Pause For 5 Seconds

It's not the same body you had as a baby, as a child, or as a teenager. You may have had bits put into it or bits cut out of it. You have scars, and wrinkles, and moles and blemishes, and sunspots. It's not the same skin you had in your youth, that's for sure. But the part of you that can notice your body never changes.

Pause For 5 Seconds

As a child, when you looked in the mirror, your reflection was very different than it is today, but the you who could notice your reflection is the same you that notices your reflection today.

Pause For 5 Seconds

Now quickly scan your body from head to toe, and notice the different feelings and sensations, and pick any feeling or sensation that captures your interest, and observe it with curiosity, noticing where it starts and stops, and how deep in it goes, and what its shape is, and its temperature. And as you notice this feeling or sensation, just be aware you're noticing, there is the feeling, and there you are noticing it.

Pause For 5 Seconds

If you can notice this feeling or sensation, you cannot be this feeling or sensation.

Pause For 5 Seconds

Your feelings and sensations change continually, sometimes you feel happy, sometimes you feel sad, sometimes you feel healthy, sometimes you feel sick, sometimes you feel stressed, sometimes relaxed, but the part of you that notices your feelings does not change.

Pause For 5 Seconds

And when you're frightened, angry, or sad in your life today, the you who can notice those feelings is the same you that could notice your feelings as a child.

Now notice the role you're playing in this moment, and as you do that, be aware you're noticing, right now, you're playing the role of a client, but your roles change continuously, at times, you're in the role of a mother/father, son/daughter, brother/sister, friend, enemy, neighbor, rival, student, teacher, citizen, customer, worker, employer, employee, and so on.

Pause For 5 Seconds

If you can notice those roles, you cannot be those roles.

Pause For 5 Seconds

And there are some roles that you will never have again, like the role of a young child.

Pause For 5 Seconds

But the you who notices your roles does not change. It's the same you that could notice your roles even when you were very young. We don't have a good name in everyday language for this part of you. I'm going to call it the observing self, but you don't have to call it that, you can call it whatever you like, and this observing self is like the sky

Every mental pathology comes from F.E.A.R.: an acronym for 4 mental processes that lead to all mental problems:

- **Fusion with your thoughts**
- **Evaluation of experience**
- **Avoidance of your experience**
- **Reason-giving for your behavior**

The healthy alternative is to A.C.T.:

- **Accept your reactions and be present**
- **Choose a valued direction**
- **Take action**

Let's now quickly overview each aspect of F.E.A.R.:

FUSION WITH YOUR THOUGHTS

As you've read in the previous lesson about cognitive defusion, when you fuse with your thoughts you're a slave to your past programming and habits such as your porn addiction. Fusing with your thoughts causes your depression, anxiety and every other kind of negative and unproductive thinking to take over. (Wilson & DuFrene, 2012)

EVALUATION OF EXPERIENCE

The human working memory is limited to about 7 chunks of information per moment. When we judge and evaluate our experience, we use up a large chunk of our brainpower for something that's completely unproductive. Additionally, if you remember the lesson about experiential avoidance, evaluating our experience turns clean pain into dirty pain. Evaluation of experience is the reason why Zebras don't get stress ulcers even though they have to fight for their lives all the time. They don't judge it as bad and don't ruminate on the 'terrible lion that hunts them', instead they just accept what's happening in the moment, let it go, and realize that what is in the moment is. The only way to change for the better is to accept the present and ACT. (Harris, 2009)

AVOIDANCE OF YOUR EXPERIENCE

Since humans judge an experience as bad or wrong, they come to the conclusion that they should avoid certain experiences. As you have read in previous lessons, experiential avoidance has been found to be the root cause behind every addiction, such as porn addiction and other behavioral problems such as procrastination. It also exacerbates seemingly unrelated pathologies such as depression, anxiety and essentially everything else. A person with anxiety becomes dysfunctional mostly because they try to avoid their anxiety. They very severely limit their ability to ACT in the world by avoiding all the situations that cause their anxiety. Similarly, a person with depression tries to avoid their depression by watching TV, drinking, using porn and other unproductive activities. (Harris, 2009)

REASON-GIVING FOR YOUR BEHAVIOR

Your mind will always give you reasons why you should use porn, and it will also give you reasons why you shouldn't use porn. What it comes down to is making the choice to use porn or not. A choice is when you act without reasons. The mind is not involved in choices. Decisions are made by your mind when you have reasons for doing what you're doing. Because you came up with reasons for and against using porn, you need to set your mind aside and simply make a choice on whether or not to use porn. Reasons will not help you here. (Wilson & DuFrene, 2012)

Now let's dissect the psychologically healthy alternative:

ACCEPT YOUR REACTIONS AND BE PRESENT

This is the skill that we've been trying to teach you for the last 8 lessons. Whatever happens in the moment happens, there's not much you can do about it. And as such, the most productive reaction towards anything that happens in your present moment experience is to accept your automatic reaction to it (to become aware of it) and be present. This will allow you to take back control from your programming and your automatic negative thoughts and habits. (Wilson & DuFrene, 2012)

CHOOSE A VALUED DIRECTION

This second step will be covered the upcoming lessons. Freedom to act in any way you want is only valuable when you know what to do with it. Acceptance and mindfulness without a valued life direction leads to passivity. Having a valued direction is what distinguishes someone who practices ACT from a hippie or a new-ager who does nothing else but meditates all day. In spiritual subcultures, there are many people who do nothing else but accept life as it is. Most of the time they don't actually achieve anything substantial in the outside world. Instead of making you a navel-gazer, I want you to be a successful at life on your own terms. To achieve this you need a clear valued-direction. (Wilson & DuFrene, 2012)

Additionally, a clear valued direction will lead you away from all unproductive activities such as using porn. When you fill up your time with something you value, you don't have time for unproductive and unfulfilling things such as porn addiction.

TAKE ACTION

In real life, your insides are just as good as what they make you do. Once you've chosen your values and learned to be mindful of your internal landscape and take back behavioral control from your mind, there's nothing keeping you from ACTing in a productive way every day. This is what will ultimately transform you into a person that people will naturally be attracted to. This is what will make you a success in life. Action. Nothing else but action. At this point, I want you to give you a short theoretical summary of all mindfulness meditations, so you'll know how different meditations, such as observing your breath, and observing sounds essentially teach the same thing.

Almost all mindfulness exercises are composed of:

- Noticing your experience as it is in the moment

- Cognitive Defusion (sometimes it's implied)
- Acceptance of your experience

So essentially if you want to conquer porn addiction and all other pathologies all you need is to do is to move from **FEAR** to **ACTion**. Nothing more. Nothing less. And to do this you just have to practice the meditations you've practiced so far in this course daily. Just schedule a time in the day when you'll listen to one of them. And just listen to one meditation every day.

EXERCISE

REWRITE YOUR STORY

Please describe in writing the key historical events that have shaped your life and have made you into what you are today. After you've written a page, please underline all the objective facts such as "I had a panic attack in middle school" then circle all the psychological reactions (thoughts, feelings, memories, sensations, urges, dispositions and so on such as "I thought I was going to die"). Then write the story again with all the underlined and circled content remaining, but with a different theme and ending. The purpose is not to prove that the original story is 'wrong' it's just an exercise that will show you how your mind works

WRITE AN OBJECTIVE STORY

Now as you did that part of the exercise, I would like you to write yet another story. Now write a story that includes only the objective facts with different psychological reactions, evaluations and judgments. Remember this particular exercise is just an opportunity to see how our minds make sense of things and what kinds of things go into a personal story. It's also a chance to notice how we get attached and invested in certain aspects of a life story when in fact there are many ways to think of things. That is not a good or bad thing, just something we want to be aware of.

LISTEN TO YOUR THOUGHTS

For the next thirty seconds, silently listen in to what your mind is saying. And if your thoughts stop, just keep listening until they start again. Then, have a pause for thirty seconds. So there you have it: there's a part of your mind that talks -The thinking self- and a part of your mind that listens- the observing self.

NOTICE HOW YOUR CONCEPTUALIZED SELF LIMITS YOU

Write out a few sentences using this template:

Because I am_____ (insert a symptom, role, or story here), I can't____(insert a valued action here).

[10]

Musturbation- The Essence of Self Destructive Thinking AKA How to Heal the Unproductive Thought Patterns That Make You Compulsively Use Porn

AS YOU HAVE LEARNED in previous chapters about cognitive fusion, external events cannot directly trigger a negative emotional experience. What they can do is to trigger a thought or belief which will trigger a negative emotional experience when you'll fuse with it. (Ellis & Ellis, 2011) The majority these pathological thoughts come from 'must' and 'should' thinking At the root of rational-emotive behavioral therapy is the truth that it's perfectly rational to have preferences and choices (such as your values) but these can become pathological when you turn these preferences into demands or 'musts'.(Ellis & Ellis, 2011)

According to REBT, thoughts have the ability to create the most significant emotional problems when you believe something **MUST** be or must not be. For example: "I must have a partner" instead of "I prefer to have a partner." (Ellis & Ellis, 2011)

The belief: "I prefer to have a good grade in this exam" will not create anxiety, even if you fuse with it, while the belief "I MUST have a good grade in this exam" will.

Do you remember our lesson about experiential avoidance? This is relevant there too. The belief that "I must never have anxiety" will create more anxiety, while the belief "I prefer not to have anxiety, but I accept it when I do" won't.

The belief "My significant other MUST not behave coldly toward me" will create resentment when occasionally, and even unintentionally, your partner will behave coldly towards you. But the belief "I find it Unpleasant when my spouse behaves coldly towards me" won't.

Whenever you hold the belief that something must or must not happen, you also hold the implied judgment that when it happens or does not happen it's awful, terrible and unbearable, which leads to experiential avoidance and the inability to be in the present moment.

THINKING IN MUSTS IS THE ESSENCE OF UNREALISTIC, IRRATIONAL AND SELF-DESTRUCTIVE THINKING.

There are three kinds of musts/irrational demands:
- Demands on oneself
- Demands on other people
- Demands on the situation (or on the universe)

Preferences almost never turn into pathology. Let's say that you have something that most people would call an 'unrealistic' goal and you hold it as a preference. Such as: "I keenly prefer to be the richest, and it's unfortunate that I'm not."

In of itself, this belief will not cause you emotional distress because it's only a preference. You will not feel disturbed about not being the richest person alive. Whenever a goal is viewed as a preference and not as a must, it motivates. But even the most menial goal, if turned into a must, can be turned into a pathology.

Let me give you an example: During my final year of my BSC in psychology program, I fully believed that I HAD TO have at least 3.5 GPA or ELSE my world would implode. This made me very anxious during every assignment and every exam, but once I took on the belief that "I prefer to have a 3.5 GPA or above, but it's not the end of the world if that doesn't happen" I became far more relaxed and calm. We call this kind of must-oriented thinking Musturbation.

MUSTURBATION WILL ALWAYS LEAD TO MASTURBATION

The mindfulness training we did so far will help you defuse from your MUSTS and at the same time it will make you more aware of your musts so you can tackle them directly with the technique you'll learn today. Both approaches, Defusion and the technique you're going to learn today, are complementary. They don't exclude one another. Well-practiced Defusion will allow you not to be controlled by your musts when they arise in your mind, and the technique you're going to learn today will allow you to change them into healthy rational thought patterns.

Awareness of your musts won't solve your irrational thought patterns. To do this, you will have to write down every must you notice in your journal and apply this technique to each and every single one. This is actually doable; we really don't have that many musts in our mind. It might seem like much but if you tackle just one must per day you'll transform your pathological thought patterns into healthy thought patterns before you know it.

In the technique you'll learn in this lesson, you'll be asked to list out the musts you'll notice thanks to the increased awareness you gained through your mindfulness practice and then dispute them one by one. You'll be essentially asked to debate with yourself.

THE THREE MINUTE THERAPY TECHNIQUE

This technique was created by Dr Michael Edelstein and is based on REBT (Rational-Emotive Behavioral Therapy) and Cognitive Behavioral Therapy. It's an easy to use technique that will take only 3 minutes to implement each time you use it. With it you'll have everything you need to bust your musts and turn them into healthy preferences. (Edelstein, 2009)

The steps required to execute it are simple.

Simply practice mindfulness daily and become more aware, through that notice whenever you hold 'must' beliefs. Write them down in your journal

And then bust them one by one using the Three Minute Therapy Technique It's that simple.

Do this every day and you'll soon turn all your unhealthy thought patterns into health thought patterns. The Three Minute Exercise Will follow a very easy to remember ABCDEF format.

The ABC model is a model that explains how situations cause your negative emotions:

Let's look at it with an example of anger:

• A(Activating event): My girlfriend didn't want to have sex with me today
• B(Irrational belief): My girlfriend MUST want to have sex with me everyday
• C(Emotional consequence): Anger

As you see it's the MUST's that makes you angry. Not the fact that your girlfriend didn't want sex with you today.

Let's look at a more relevant example that illustrates how 'musts' also relate to the concept of experiential avoidance which you have learned previously:

- **A(Activating EVENT):** You feel stressed by doing a chore.
- **B (Irrational belief):** I MUST NOT feel STRESSED.
- **C (Emotional consequence):** You feel stressed about your stress.

At this point it's important to note that "hate to's" are nothing more but musts.
Let's now look how this will progress:

- **A (Activating event):** Feeling stressed about stress.
- **B (Irrational belief):** I HAVE TO ELEVIATE MY STRESS. I HAVE TO GET RID OF THIS EMOTION.
- **C (Consequence):** "I'll use porn to quickly alleviate my stress.

MUST's created these negative behavioral and emotional responses. But how do we turn musts into preferences? It's simple, we do it by doing "D", Dispute them.
This involves asking "What's the evidence for my MUST?"
Or in our example: "Why must my girlfriend give me sex every day?"
The correct response is often surprising: There's really no evidence for this must or any MUST. No reason exists that your girlfriend MUSTS do other than that she does, however desirable you might find it if she did. So now we can move on to "E" – Effective New Thinking: "I would prefer it if my girlfriend had sex with me every day, but I can survive quite well if she doesn't"
It's true that you find it unpleasant that your girlfriend won't have sex with you every day, and that you would like it better if she did. But

the universe is not created so that people always do what you'd prefer them to do. Therefore it's unrealistic to expect this, and to demand that it MUST occur.

Additionally, whenever you demand that something must occur you create an implied thought that something terrible will happen if it doesn't occur. People tend to unconsciously think that if they won't get their musts that something equivalent to the end of the universe will happen. They express this by using words such as "awful", "appalling", "dreadful", or "horrible". But the truth is that although you dislike the fact that your girlfriend won't have sex with you, you can survive quite well without having sex with your girlfriend today.

When you replace your B (Your irrational demand that your girlfriend MUST have sex with you) with an E (A rational preference for daily sex) you'll begin to experience "F", A new feeling

In this case you'll feel disappointment but not anger.

This technique is simple. But mastery of it requires continuous daily practice.

That's why you'll be asked to do it every day in your journal from now on.

In a way this exercise just like your daily meditation and other questions in your journal should become a daily practice. They are like brushing your teeth. Imagine you've been brushing your teeth for a year and then you go to a dentist and he says "Your teeth are healthy" will you stop brushing your teeth just because of that? If you did your teeth would quickly become unhealthy. It's the same with the techniques found here. You have to make them a daily practice. It doesn't take much to do so. And the benefits don't only relate to quitting porn addiction.

Once you develop mindfulness skills and bust your musts this will:

• 	Alleviate all of your negative emotions, including depression and anxiety

- Give you greater behavioral control. You'll procrastinate less, and be more able to accomplish your goals.
- You will become more productive.
- You'll be more immune to all other addictions, not only porn.
- You'll learn to think clearly and make more appropriate decisions.
- Because of the mind-body connection, your physical health will increase.

As you can see there are numerous benefits to practicing the mindfulness and other exercises found in the NoPorn Plan indefinitely. The NoPorn Plan is designed to not only help you with your porn addiction but give you a system of continuous self-development which you'll be able to practice for the rest of your life.

And remember you'll be able to apply this three minute therapy technique not only to porn-related problems, but to all of your problems. We'll just focus on porn-related problems in this book, because this is the NoPorn Plan.

Many people think that therapy can 'cure' them. No psychotherapy can do that. The only thing that psychotherapy can do is to give you tools and you'll be then responsible for using them on your own. Sobriety from porn, addiction, and psychological health overall takes consistent work equivalent to brushing your teeth or doing pushups. We made the NoPornPlan to provide you with the assortment of effective tools and teachings for you to scrub the porn influence off and to train yourself to be resilient against it and life's many hurdles.

MUSTS CAN ALSO POWER-UP YOUR RELAPSES

Let's imagine you've relapsed on porn and you have one of these irrational thought patterns:

"I must recover quickly without any relapses."

This belief will lead to a guilt trip and make you more prone to relapsing on porn in the future.

Let's debunk this belief using **ABCDEF**.

- **A** - Activating Event - I relapsed to porn
- **B** - Irrational belief – I must recover quickly without any relapses.
- **C** - (Consequence of that belief) – I beat myself up and guilt trip myself, which makes me relapse again.
- **D** - (Dispute)

1. -No law carved in stone states that I MUST;
2. -It's typically human and understandable that I would upset myself about a setback;
3. -I can recover slowly;
4. -It's just a hassle, not a horror;
5. -I'm not worthless because I screw up;
6. -If I don't recover quickly, I can learn from my mistakes and eventually do better at recovering;
7. -Recovering slowly means that success takes longer. It doesn't mean total failure;
8. -One failure doesn't mean total failure, or that I'll never succeed;
9. -This just means I had better work harder at it next time;
10. -This assumes that I MUST be porn free-- but, although I would like to be porn free, I don't HAVE to be;
11. -I can stand slow recoveries, although I don't like them;
12. -Reality is reality, not what I think it MUST be;
13. -If I pressure myself to always recover quickly, that will tend to make it more difficult to do so;
14. -Being an imperfect human, like all humans, I will sometimes act imperfectly.

E- Effective new thinking- While I would prefer to recover quickly without any relapses at all, it's not terrible if I get an occasional relapse and then set myself back on the road towards recovery.

F- New Feeling-Disappointment, but not self-defeat.

After completing these ABCDEFs in your journal. You might find it helpful to re-read your journal entries. Sometimes we forget about the irrationality of our pathological thought patterns, and being reminded about the traps your mind has for you helps a lot. The cognitive defusion skills you've learned in the previous lessons will also help. They'll make not only identifying irrational thought patterns easier, but they'll also take away a lot of the control your irrational thought patterns have over you, making it easier for you to change them.

EXERCISE

Can You think of any irrational thoughts you might be having? In relation to porn?

Try to debunk them using the ABCDEF procedure outlined in this lesson.

Tackling Problematic Thought Patterns

While musts are the main culprits, there are other destructive thought patterns you can bust using ABCDEF.

For example:

COMPARISONS AND EVALUATIONS – Unproductive thought patterns compare things to one another. They judge things as better or worse, usually the past or the future is judged as 'better' and the now as 'worse'.

CONFUSED THINKING – Some thoughts are especially complicated. The most dangerous ones are the ones that say that this or that particular problem has to be fixed before you can do something productive.

BUT's – This one is self-explanatory if you read these examples:

If I don't quit porn I'll never have a healthy sexual life, but I don't know if I can stop.

I'd like to have an intimate relationship, but first I need to lose a significant amount of weight. Having a job is a top priority for me, but until I get this back pain problem solved, that's just not an option for me.

In a nutshell: BUT's are just excuses to not get something done.

If only's – If only I had more self-control, then I would quit porn.

If I felt confident enough, then I would be successful.

If I lost enough weight, then I could have a relationship.

If I didn't have to worry about money, my life would be much happier.

If my pain goes away, then I will be able to go back to work.

They try to prove they're right. They try very hard to solve an internal problem. And as you've learned in previous lessons trying to solve internal problems using external techniques is counterproductive.

When you think of your past, do you think of them in descriptive terms or as explanations? "I masturbated for 6 hours yesterday because I was so much stressed and couldn't handle it." "I relapsed on weight gain porn because I was overwhelmed and was afraid." By giving reasons to your counterproductive behaviors. You're rationalizing it.

BLACK AND WHITE THINKING: WHY AFFIRMATIONS DON'T WORK

Affirmations don't work for several reasons. First and foremost, you state something that's obviously false at the current time, which creates a feeling of incongruence in your mind. When you say "I'm thin" while weighing 600 pounds your mind knows that's not true and will immediately respond with "No. You're not. You're fat", which will take the power away from your affirmation.

At the same time hidden deeply in each affirmation, there's an implication of a MUST. For example, when you say "I am porn free and I will be porn free forever" you're essentially creating a "Must". "I must be porn free."

So what's the alternative?

THE HEALTHY ALTERNATIVE TO AN AFFIRMATION IS A CHOICE

Instead of saying: "I'll never masturbate to porn" (which creates a MUST. "I must never masturbate to porn.") You can choose to say: "I choose to be porn free." or "I choose not to masturbate to porn."

This is an important distinction and we'll use an affirmation like this in yet another relapse prevention technique which we'll teach you in the module after the next.

Let's now use Three Minute Therapy to disprove some of the most common thoughts held by porn addicts.

These are:

- "I MUST quit porn quickly."
- "Life should be more fun."
- "I must be porn free, or else I'm less of a person."
- "If I start to feel bored or dissatisfied, I MUST feel better right away."
- "Other people can overcome their addiction, but not me."

- "It's not only hard to stop the addiction' but it's too hard."
- "It shouldn't be hard, and it definitively shouldn't be this hard."
- "I deserve to have it easier. I deserve to give up porn without any effort whatsoever."
- "I should be able to get away with this. Other people might of course destroy their sexuality with porn. But not me. For me it should be just an easy past time."
- "It's bad to be deprived. I shouldn't deprive myself of pleasure. I can't stand deprivation, and I certainly can't stand frustration and pain."
- "It will be easier to stop tomorrow. I'll just wait for tomorrow then I'll quit porn. Why do I have to quit porn now if I can just wait for tomorrow when it will be easier? I can wait indefinitely..."
- "It's my nature to compulsively desire porn. I was born a porn user and that's my nature. I should use porn."
- "I MUST have this immediate gratification. Not only I like it and desire it. But I MUST have this immediate gratification."
- "Life is to unexciting and boring if I stop using porn, therefore I MUST go on and do porn."
- "If I stop using porn I'll feel anxious, and I can't bear anxiety, and as such I must use porn."
- "There must be a magical easy way to stop using porn, and I'll wait for it."
- "I know other people change and maybe when I was young I could do so, but now I'm too old to stop using porn."

All of these stories boil down to one thing: "The world should be easier than it is and I can't bear it when it isn't. So I'll go on and numb myself with porn to be able to bear life."

The third set of destructive stories/thoughts could be grouped into 'hostility', 'anger' or putting others down.

"You shouldn't make me stop using porn you bastard! You should allow me. In fact you should encourage me to go on wasting my life on porn. But you're making me stop. How awful!"

"The world is against me if I have to give up this pleasure. This horrible world... How could it be that way? I can't stand this world! Do I really have to stop using porn?"

"You should make things easier for me. You should figure out how to make me quit porn without any involvement on my part. What you're doing so far is not good enough because I still can use porn if I really try

THOUGHTS ABOUT HAVING THE SYMPTOMS

Once you're addicted, you're addicted. It's undeniable if you masturbate for 6 hours per day and if you have 1TB of porn on your hard drive. And as such, you'll develop the thought that you're no good. Once you develop the story that you're no good, you might fuse with it. When you fuse with it, you actually believe you're no good. How can someone who's fundamentally no good quit porn addiction, even with the help of the NoPorn Plan?

"If I'll know how I got this way, my symptoms will disappear. So I'll rather go to psychoanalysis for 40 years and that's the way to get rid of these symptoms."

"The NoPorn plan should make me stop even if I don't do any of the exercises, and don't practice meditations every day. What the hell do they expect? I paid them for their dammed book and they actually expect me to go through and do the exercises it to get a result? Preposterous!"

"I've realized that there's really no way to cure an addiction without effort or work, and that's HARD. And it's TOO HARD. "

Cognitive defusion will also help you to take away the power of these irrational thoughts. Once you identify any of these thoughts in yourself. You can tackle them directly using REBT.

Let me give you some examples:

A-ACTIVATING EVENT: FEELING STRESSED OR AGITATED OR SEEING A SEXUAL PICTURE ON A BILLBOARD.

B-IRRATIONAL BELIEF: "I MUST USE PORN."

C-CONSEQUENCE: USING PORN: "ISN'T IT AWFUL THAT I CAN'T MASTURBATE TO PORN WHEN I WANT WITHOUT HURTING MY SEXUALITY? I CAN'T STAND THIS PAIN OF GIVING UP THIS ADDICTION... THE PAIN SHOULDN'T BE THIS WAY, AND THE WORLD SHOULDN'T BE THIS WAY. AND IF I DON'T DO THIS CORRECTLY I'M NO GOOD. AND IF THE NoPorn PLAN WON'T HELP ME OVERCOME MY LIFELONG ADDICTION WITHOUT ANY EFFORT ON MY PART THEN IT'S NO GOOD."

D-DISPUTING: WHY IS IT TOO HARD TO GIVE UP PORN?

The correct answer is: It isn't. It's only hard. Nothing is "too hard". Because "too hard" actually means that it must not be that hard, it must be easier, and it must come to me with minimal pain and minimal real effort. Where's the evidence that I HAVE TO get over this addiction without much pain, without much hassle? The answer is of course there's no reason why it must not be hard. Let's go over another common irrational beliefs our addicted selves have:

"I MUST masturbate to porn. I must have porn. I must masturbate."
Dispute: Why MUST you watch porn?
Sample answer: Because I like it, because I want it.

But why MUST you have what you want?
Sample answer: Because I want it.

Do you really want it? Do you want the results you're getting out of using it? Why must you have it? If you persist with this you'll realize that there's never a reason for a must. The thought behind it always is: "It would be nice if I could masturbate for 6 hours per day with no impact on my productivity, but it's not this way. It's awful to be deprived of porn."
Dispute: Where's the evidence that it's awful to be deprived from porn? It's awful because it's unpleasant.
"You're saying I'm not allowed any porn for the rest of my life?"

Well maybe if your addiction escalates to masturbating 6 hours per day, you are better off abstaining from porn for the rest of your life. And then you might think: "But that's awful! Horrible!"
Then we say: Prove it.
You might say how inconvenient it is. How unpleasant it is. How distasteful it is. But you'll never find a reason for awfulness, because awfulness means it's totally obnoxious that you don't get to watch porn. And it's obviously not totally awful; No one has ever died for not using porn.
Awful means it's not only obnoxious to not to use porn, but it's unpleasant to do so. Could you prove it? It is truly unpleasant not to use porn at this point in your addiction. But isn't it worse to have all of the problems associated with compulsive porn use? Quitting porn is not awful, is only uncomfortable. If you could prove it would be horrific for one to not use porn, I'd want to hear that reasoning. As of yet though, no one has ever proven that abstaining from porn was pure horror.

"I can't stand giving up pornography."

Dispute: Why can't you stand it? It's an interesting hypothesis. Prove it.

You might answer: "I'll be anxious."

Why can't you stand being anxious?

You say: "Because I'll get more anxious."

If you are unable to willingly be with that emotion, you will be. But why can't you stand to be more anxious? If you practice your ability to be willing enough through the daily practice of the mindfulness exercises found in here, you'll find that you can stand any emotion that you will ever experience. If someone literally rips you into shreds, you'll be able to 'stand it' till you die.

The view that 'I'm not supposed to stand it' is irrational. You're not supposed to like it, but you can choose to be willingly with it. Any thought that tells you 'you can't bear it' is irrational. Because if anything, that's the one thing you'll be always able to do once you're train your mindfulness muscles.

Another irrational belief is: "If the world treats me this way and makes it so unpleasant that I have to give up porn the world shouldn't be that way. It's a horrible world. It must not be that way."

Let's suppose that the world is horrible. It has taxes, you have to wake up in the morning to work and do many other things you don't enjoy. Let's suppose that the world is obnoxious. Why must it not be that way?

Why must you spend your time changing the world if you can't change it by doing so? Instead of working on your addictions to change yourself?

You can hate the world and other people, or you can realize that this won't help you ultimately make your life better.

All these musts. All these shoulds. All these "I can't stand this" are simply unproductive.

A good philosophy you can use for quitting porn is:

I may find it pretty uncomfortable, and I might find it strange to meditate every day and to write a journal every day. I will always find it uncomfortable, but I will find it more uncomfortable if I don't do these things and relapse to porn.

[11]

Learn a Technique That Will Curb Your Porn Cravings: Accupressure Desensitization

I have to admit that **Acupressure Desensitization** is not completely new. It's a modification of **EFT (Emotional Freedom Technique)**, which itself is a modification of **TFT (Thought field therapy)**. I learned EFT when I was 15, and practiced it every day since. I'm now 25, and have 10 years of experience of using this technique.

However, I found that I needed to eliminate a lot of confusion and frustration I experienced with the original EFT technique, so I created **Acupressure Desensitization**.

THE EMOTIONAL FREEDOM TECHNIQUE, ITS HISTORY, AND WHY I CREATED MY OWN TECHNIQUE

Although I've found that EFT works, as well as numerous other studies, (Feinstein, 2008) I am fully opposed all of the pseudoscientific theories presented in nearly all EFT and TFT books.(Craig, 2011; Mountrose, Mountrose, & Holistic Communications, 2005)

The biggest problem I have with these other books is that their explanation of EFT heavily relies on mysticism.

The main theory they present is that all psychological problems are caused by a 'disruption of the body's energy system'. That energy system is poorly defined and you're asked to accept it as is, leaving you with far more questions than results. Also, because of its over-reliance on this pseudoscientific energetic explanation, these books generally don't adequately explain how EFT works, keeping you from utilizing this technique for your own custom needs.

I've personally spent years trying to "de-code" this mysticism language to make the most of what EFT had to offer. For your benefit, I refuse to add any unnecessary mysticism to this technique. In fact, there's no need to bring up the ancient energy metaphor because it's just a metaphor, even though most 'energy therapy' practitioners treat it as fact.

With the mystic lingo aside, there is actual proof that EFT works and its efficacy can be fully explained by modern psychology, without pseudoscientific explanations about energies, polarities or other magical things.

ACUPRESSURE DESENSITIZATION IS ESSENTIALLY EFT WITHOUT THE B.S.

Life is confusing enough without putting filler into a self-help technique. Unlike EFT, Acupressure Desensitization fully disregards the notion of energies because this is just a metaphor for internal experiences. Studies have shown that when uninformed natives or children try to explain something biological without any knowledge of it, they tend to use 'energy' explanations. It's simply a metaphor that resonates with us as a species and was used for over millennia by our forefathers because they simply didn't know any better, and had to explain internal phenomenon somehow. Now that we have modern medicine and science, this kind of explanation is not the best one for if you are looking for results you can use in your daily life.

HOW AND WHY ACUPRESSURE DESENSITIZATION WORKS

Before I go into theoretical details let me explain to you very quickly how AD is done so you'll know what I'm talking about.
AD In a Nutshell:

• First, you rate the distress behind whatever you're desensitizing on the **Subjective Unit Of Distress** scale from 1- 10 so you'll know where you're at and can measure your improvement.

• Next, you affirm your willingness to be present with the problem you're working on with the **Setup Phrase**.

• Then you stimulate acupoints while thinking of the problem. You remind yourself of the problem using a very specific **Acupressure Desensitization Affirmation**.

• You rate yourself again and see if there was improvement.

• You repeat steps 1-4 until you experience no distress/reaction to the thing you've picked in step 1.

That's it. It's a very simple technique that will allow you to:

• Lower your porn craving as it arises (desensitize it)

• Lower the emotional charge of any memory you use AD on, making it far easier to defuse from it.

• Lower the emotional charge of any negative belief you might have, making it far easier to defuse from it.

• Lower the emotional charge of any sexual fantasy or urge, making it far easier to defuse from it.

• Lower the emotional charge of anything else, making it far easier to defuse from it.

Whenever you find that a memory or thought is too emotionally charged for you to easily defuse from it, you'll simply use AD on it, and then once its charge is lowered you'll be able to defuse from it easily.

It's really a no-nonsense technique that will aid your journal to self-improvement. It's an ideal complement to everything else you've learned in the Mindfulness Skills section.

Let's now look under the hood of AD and see why it works.

WHAT THE HELL DO ACUPRESSURE POINTS HAVE TO DO WITH DESENSITIZING EMOTIONS?

EFT originally postulated that 'all negative emotions are caused by disruptions in the body's energy system'. If you have any scientific background at all, you might think that this is the single most pseudoscientific statement you've ever heard.

And you'd be correct.

Acupressure can be explained in way that doesn't refer to an esoteric system of energies at all. Acupoints are something that's actually proven by science; they are simply places on our skin with greater than average electromagnetic conductivity.

It also has been directly proven that stimulating acupoints in any way sends relaxation signals to our brain. Scientists have actually looked at the brain response during acupoint stimulation and it has been shown that stimulating acupoints sends deactivating signals to the limbic system, the part of our brain that's responsible for craving and emotions.

So when you think of something upsetting, your limbic system gets activated. By stimulating your acupoints by tapping, you're sending signals to your brain to deactivate them. So you get two conflicting signals which cancel each other out. This is a proven and widely observed phenomenon in psychology. That's all that Acupressure Desensitization does.

In reality, EFT is nothing but an upgraded form of systematic desensitization.

If you have ever read anything about psychology before, you might have heard about systematic desensitization. Systematic desensitization is a therapy which uses multiple exposures to an uncomfortable stimulus or memory in order to take away its emotional power. (Wenrich, Dawley, & General, 1976)

THERE ARE THREE STEPS IN THE SELF-ADMINISTERED SYSTEMATIC DESENSITIZATION PROCEDURE:

Procedure:
- 1: Relaxation
- 2: Constructing an anxiety hierarchy (Imaging specific anxiety events and rating them in intensity)
- 3: Pairing relaxation with the situations described in your anxiety hierarchy

Acupressure desensitization uses acupressure stimulation as a vector of relaxation and as such acupressure Desensitization is nothing more but an upgraded version of systematic desensitization. It's upgraded in the following ways:

1. In normal systematic desensitization, you're required to experience your negative emotion and craving in full. In Acupressure Desensitization, you're technically keeping it in mind through the Acupressure Desensitization Affirmation (or the reminder phrase in EFT) but at the same time you don't have to emotionally recall your problem or negative memory. Tapping essentially distracts your

mind enough so that you're not overwhelmed by negative emotions, while the Acupressure Desensitization Affirmation (the reminder phrase) keeps your problem in mind sufficiently for it to be desensitized through exposure and through tapping. To put it differently, your working memory is taxed by tapping, while your problem is still kept in awareness through the Acupressure Desensitization Affirmation, which allows you to desensitize your emotional problems without necessarily experiencing them fully. It's important to note that one can be re-traumatized if one re-experiences overwhelming negative emotions. The Acupressure Desensitization Affirmation avoids this and allows you to use systematic desensitization in an easy way on your own without necessarily being guided by anyone else. Your working memory has a storage system called the 'phonological loop' in cognitive psychology and when you're repeating your reminder phrase either out loud or in your mind, you're storing your problem in your working memory without necessarily re-experiencing it, which allows you to desensitize from it without re-experiencing it.

2. In normal systematic desensitization, you're told to relax by listening to a progressive relaxation recording, not unlike some of the guided meditations we have here. In this program, you relax by tapping acupressure points. With this you can tell your brain to relax at the exact same time as you're recalling your emotional problem. This is far more powerful and desensitizes (discharges) the emotional problem far quicker.

But just because Acupressure Desensitization doesn't claim to do anything 'magic' like EFT does, it doesn't mean it's any less powerful. You can use it to desensitize any SPECIFIC emotion, belief or thought that you find hard to defuse from. You'll find that it's a very useful supplement to your Mindfulness Skills Training.

There are several different ways you can use AD to work through your issues. The most straightforward is simply to pick a specific issue (as specific as possible) and use it as the AD affirmation.

LET'S NOW LOOK MORE CLOSELY AT THE DIFFERENT STEPS OF ACUPRESSURE DESENSITIZATION

Before You do anything rate yourself using the Subjective Units Of distress

The first thing you do when you do Acupressure Desensitization is that you measure your Subjective Units of Distress. You essentially measure the intensity of the specific problem you're working on a scale of 1- 10. If you're using this on physical pain such as a headache you would measure the intensity of your headache on the scale of 1-10. If you were working on a specific emotional problem such as a phobia, like for example "fear of spiders" you would measure the intensity of your fear of spiders on a scale of 1-10. If you were working on a specific craving, such as the craving for porn, you would measure the craving for porn on a scale of 1-10. 1 being no craving and 10 being the strongest craving you've ever experienced.

2. The Set up Phrase: The step-up phrase is designed to be an affirmation of your acceptance and commitment to get over the problem. It puts you into the correct frame of mind to work on your problem using Acupressure Desensitization.

The original set up phrase in the Emotional Freedom Technique was:

"Even though I have <name of problem>, I deeply and completely love and accept myself."

All it is an affirmation of your willingness to be present with the problem and accept yourself as you are in the present moment. You can modify it so it will sound more natural for you. For example:

"Even though I have <name of the problem you work on>, I choose to accept myself and be present with it."

"Even though I have <name of the problem you're working on>, I accept and love myself."

"Even though I <name of the problem you're working on>, I choose to be present with it and do my best to act in a value-based way."

"Even though I <name of the problem you're working on>, I choose to be the ultimate me."

"Even though I <name of the problem you're working on>, I am okay."

Now more deeper examples:

"Even though I'm afraid of spiders, I'm okay."

"Even though I really crave porn right now, I choose to be present with it and do my best to act in a value-based way."

"Even though I have this deep craving for porn, I deeply and completely accept my myself."

"Even though I have this deep craving for porn, I love and accept myself."

"Even though I have this deep craving for porn, I'm okay."

"Even though I have this deep craving for porn, I choose to be present with it."

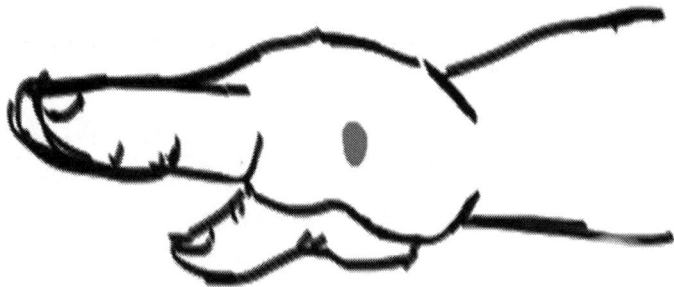

You get the idea. The idea is to communicate that even though you have this problem, you accept yourself as you are and you choose to be present with your problem. Some people feel uncomfortable with saying the word' love' because it sounds weird, and you really don't have to. The original EFT creators were really into the whole New - Age hippie shtick of 'love for all', and as such they used the word because they liked it. You don't have to use it. The whole point of the set up phrase is to communicate that even though you've got the problem, you accept yourself and your current state. That's it. The specific phrasing doesn't matter. If you can come up with your own version of it, use it. The only requirement is that it contains both an acceptance and an exposure statement.

You say this set up phrase 3 times out loud or silently in your mind while tapping on the 'karate chop point'. Which is located on the side of your hand, I.e. the part of your hand you' would use to deliver a karate chop. There's really nothing special about this point other than the fact that it's large and will allow you to very easily tap or massage it while repeating this affirmation 3 times. Alternatively you can put your hand on your chest and take a few deep breaths after repeating each affirmation. The idea is to simply relax by stimulating your acupuncture points while repeating this affirmation.

By reminding yourself to be willingly present with your problem, the set-up phrase eliminates any unconscious self-sabotage that might be present during your Acupressure Desensitization session.

After this you'll have to come up with your Acupuncture Desensitization Affirmation.

THE ACUPRESSURE DESENSITIZATION AFFIRMATION

It's important for your Acupressure Desensitization Phrase to be as specific as possible. You want to create something that your mind can very easily imagine, so that it can be stored in your working memory as you stimulate your acupressure points.

For example, let's say that your problem is that you feel stressed during tests, and you have a very big test coming up tomorrow. An example of Acupressure Desensitization Affirmation could be "That test" or "The test I have to take tomorrow". This is a specific phrase because it conjures a very specific image in your mind which you can desensitize by stimulating your acupressure points.

In Acupressure Desensitization, it's important for your Acupressure Desensitization Affirmation to be as specific as possible. That's because we aim to put a very specific picture into your working memory so that we can desensitize it. We need to desensitize specific thoughts. After repetitions of AD, the desensitization effect will generalize into numerous other memories and thoughts.

Desensitization however doesn't work on ambiguous or broad problems such as 'self-esteem', 'depression', or 'performance problems'. We have a different technique for that called the Mindful Acupressure Therapy which we will teach you in the last lesson, but for now you need some practice with Acupressure Desensitization.

For acupressure desensitization to work you have to tune into the events that contributed to your global problem and desensitize them one by one. Both EFT and acupressure desensitization chunk down problems into smaller pieces called aspects. When you desensitize them one by one, slowly but surely the emotional pattern underlying these problems will lose its power and you'll have a much easier time defusing from all of the beliefs, thoughts and emotions that fuel your problem, in this case, porn addiction.

Each problem can be chunked down and the strongest emotional charge will be in only one of the chunks. More often than not, you'll be able to create a Still Frame Picture of that chunk so you'll be able to desensitize that aspect of your problem that way.

Remember, your problems are caused by thoughts and beliefs you fuse with. Acupressure Desensitization helps you take the emotional charge away from these thoughts and beliefs, which will make it easier for you to defuse from them. You'll still need to practice mindfulness to do that, but it will be easier.

Here are some questions that will allow you to identify some aspects to tap to:

Does the problem that's bothering you remind you of any events in your childhood? Tune into your body and feel your feelings. Then travel back in time to the first time in your life you ever felt that same sensation.

What's the worst similar experience you ever had? If you were writing your autobiography, what chapter would you prefer to delete, as though it had never happened to you?

Now you'll essentially tap each point of either the full **AD** (described below) while repeating the Acupressure Desensitization Affirmation to yourself once at each point.

YOU CAN USE A STILL FRAME PICTURE AS AN ALTERNATIVE TO THE ACUPRESSURE DESENSITIZATION AFFIRMATION.

Remember the whole point of the Acupressure Desensitization Affirmation is to keep the problem in mind in a comfortable way while stimulating your acupressure points. As an alternative to this, you could also create a picture in your mind of the event you're desensitizing and 'freeze it' in time. A picture that's frozen in this way has much less emotional significance and can also be used as a reminder. In this case, you would just hold this still frame picture. It's very simple to create one.

- Simply think of the problem you want to work on. Think of it as a movie.
- Pick one 'picture' from that problem. One frozen in place picture.
- Now think of that picture while stimulating your acupoints.

It's that simple.

The Acupoints and Their Stimulation

Tap on all the points shown in acupressure desensitization while saying your Acupressure Desensitization Affirmation out loud or in your mind.

The order of how you do it does not matter at all. But since it's easier to remember, most people stimulate from top to bottom.

So you would start in this order:

You might now ask. "Why do we have to stimulate all of these acupresure points if they all do the same thing? (Sending relaxation signals to our brain) Well moving from point to point is yet another factor that helps you relax. When you have a long list of points, you have a lot of movements from point to point. But for people who'll prefer to only use a smaller amount of points we have prepared alternative sequences:

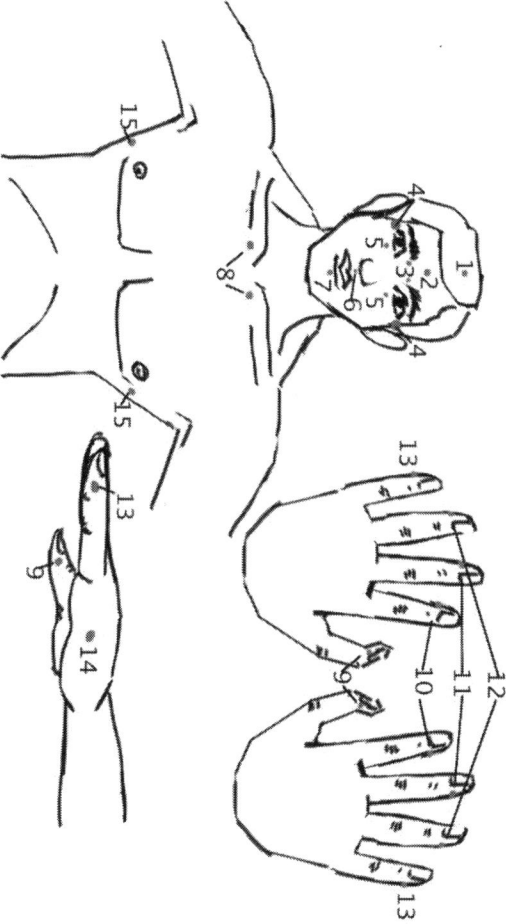

Acupressure Desensitization Points

1. **Top Of The Head:** The highest point on the top of your head.

2. **Third Eye Point:** In the center of your forehead.

3. **Start Of The Eyebrow:** Where the bone behind your eyebrow turns into the bridge of your nose.

4. **Corner Of The Eye:** On the bone in the corner of your eye.

5. **Under The Eye:** On the bone just below your eye, in line with your pupil if you look straight ahead.

6. **Under The Nose:** Between your nose and your upper lip.

7. **Under The Mouth:** In the indentation between your chin and your lower lip.

8. **Under The Collarbone:** In the angle formed by your collarbone and the breastbone.

9. **Thumb:** All finger points are on the side of the finger, in line with the nail bed.

10. **Index Finger**

11. **Middle Finger**

12. **Ring Finger**

13. **Little Finger**

14. **Karate Chop Point:** on the side of your hand, roughly in line with your life line.

You can stimulate your acupressure points any way you like.

Most people who write about EFT like it because it's very formulaic and since they use esoteric-mumbo-jumbo to explain it ("Energies','Thought-fields","Chakras")they don't really understand how, and why it this technique works and as such they don't know how to modify it. That's why almost every EFT/TFT book out there will tell you to tap, because that's what they read in their manual, and they are essentially just rewriting it.

In here you'll get better than this: You'll learn how and why Acupressure Desensitization (OR "Emotional Freedom Technique", if

you want to use the popular, less scientific name for it) works. With this, you'll be able to see through every bit of B.S. advice in this sub-field of psychotherapy and you'll be able to adjust this technique for your own needs.

For example, you'll understand that it <u>really doesn't matter</u> how you'll stimulate your acupressure points. Tapping is an easy way to do it, but it's not the only way. Other ways you can stimulate your acupressure points include but are not limited to:

- Lightly press into them and breathing deeply: This is actually the way I usually practice it.
- Massaging them.
- Applying rhythmic pressure into them. It's like tapping without taking your fingers away from the point you're 'tapping'.

These methods are especially useful when you try to use the technique that I'll teach you in the next lesson.

LET'S NOW COMBINE THE ELEMENTS TOGETHER INTO ACUPRESSURE DESENSITIZATION

1. State your emotional problem as specifically as possible.
2. Rate the intensity of your problem on a 1-10 scale. This is called your SUD.
3. State your problem in a way that's as specific as possible. Say or think the setup phrase either while tapping the karate chop point or while holding down the center of your chest and taking a deep breath. Repeat the setup phrase 3 times.
4. Create an Acupressure Desensitization Affirmation or a Still Frame Picture, and either tap for about seven times on each of the points of the AD Sequence or stimulate the acupoints in a different

way while saying/thinking the **AD** affirmation on each point or keeping the Still Frame Picture in mind.

5. Rate the intensity of the problem again. If it's not "0" proceed to step 6.

6. Repeat the sequence again, while modify your setup phrase with "Even though I still have some of this problem..." and your Acupressure Desensitization phrase with "the remaining problem". For example, if it was a fear of tests, the reminder phrase would be "The remaining fear of tests".

That's all there is to it.

TELL THE STORY TECHNIQUE

AD is great at eliminating emotional intensity but only when it's used on an actual concrete and specific event such as "John yelled at me in the meeting" or "my craving to masturbate to feet porn" rather than a general statement such as "My porn addiction".

You essentially picture your problem as it was a movie (if you're doing it in your mind) or a story (If you're doing it in writing or speaking out loud) and go through it scene by scene. Whenever you reach part of the movie/story that has an emotional charge. You use the scene as an AD Affirmation

Now let's go through a no-porn related example. Let's say that you had the general problem of 'mistrust of strangers'. If you stimulated your acupoints using the AD affirmation "mistrust of strangers' you wouldn't have anything specific to desensitize and as such the technique wouldn't work. Instead you'd focus on a specific event. By discharging emotional charge from your live events it will eventually generalize and you'll have an easier time to defuse from them.

So to use the Tell The Story technique for 'mistrust of strangers' you'd have to pick a specific event and make a movie or a story out of it.

1.   In the first part of the Tell The Story technique you'd give your movie a title. Here it could be called "The Bullies" if we picked a memory of when we were bullied at school which we identified as related to our mistrust of strangers.

2.   Then you would rate your degree of emotional distress around the title. Not the movie itself. Rate it from a scale of 1-10. Write down your movie title and your number.

3.   Work the movie title into the Setup phrase of acupressure desensitization. It might sound something like this "Even though [insert movie title here], I accept myself" or "Even though I experienced[insert movie title here], I accept myself Now go through the whole AD sequence until the distress level for the title reaches 1 or 0.

4.   Then think of a neutral point before the bad events in the movie/story began to take place. For example it could be walking home from school, before bullies saw you. Once you've identified the neutral point of your story. Start running the movie through your mind, until you reach a point where the emotional intensity rises. In this example it would be the point in which you saw bullies.

5.   Stop at this point. And rate the intensity of that emotional experience. And perform a round of AD on that scene. For example "Even though I saw the bullies turn toward me, I deeply accept myself" then repeat AD until your intensity reaches 1 or 0.

6.   Now again rewind your movie to the neutral point or if you're doing it out loud or in writing start telling the story from the beginning and again stop at the point where you're getting emotional. Use that point of the story/movie to create a new AD affirmation and use it to conduct another round of AD.

7.   Repeat this until you've done AD on all emotional parts of the story/movie and you're able to tell the story without a negative emotional reaction.

8.   Once you're able to do that tell the story again just in more detail if you opted for it to be an internal movie try to make it more vivid. See if there's a negative emotional response. If there is. Desensitize it using **AD**. Repeat this process until the scene is completely cleared

Once you clear a few events like this you'll see that your overall behavioral pattern will fade. There are probably about 30-40 events that create memories that contribute to your porn addiction. Desensitizing them using **AD** will allow you to more easily defuse from your addictive urges, as they'll have a smaller emotional charge. Later on in this chapter you'll be asked to identify specific aspects and events related to your porn addiction on which you'll use **AD** on. Then you'll be asked to do this every day in your journal. This way you'll desensitize one event or memory a day.

Remember: The point of all this is to desensitize memories so that you'll be able to defuse from them when they come up in real life. The words that you say in **AD** are not that important. It's all about getting in touch with your emotions and desensitizing them through tapping.
There's also an exception to the rule of being specific. When a memory has too much emotional charge to even think about it it's useful to dissociate from it by picking a generalized statement such as "the lake incident" as your **AD** affirmation.

HOW TO USE ACUPRESSURE DESENSITIZATION WHEN YOU'RE STRESSED OR EXPERIENCE THE URGE TO USE PORN, WITHOUT ANYONE KNOWING YOU'RE DOING IT

Let's face it. EFT, and even acupressure desensitization looks strange in action. You can't really be expected to do something like that in public. But there is a way to do acupressure desensitization without looking as if you're having an OCD tik fit.

I call this technique PAD. This stands for Pocket acupressure desensitization.

Did you notice that there are five points on your hand and you can stimulate them all using in one hand? Well it truth is that most of the time that's really all you need for acupressure desensitization. Sometimes it helps to stimulate more points, but that's not because you're stimulating more 'energy channels'. It's simply because stimulating a greater amount of points contains a greater amount of novel stimulation which allows you to stay with your emotional experience for a longer period of time. It also inevitably prolongs the process, which in turn makes it 'work better' because you're simply doing Acupressure Desensitization for longer.

But really you can just do it with your hands. And to gain maximum benefits you can do it with both of your hands. Here's how to do it step by step, you can get a visualized version of this exercise at http://nopornplan.com

1.   With your left hand, press your left hand index finger tip into the side of your left hand thumb repeat the Acupressure Desensitization Affirmation in your mind, and then take a deep breath while thinking about it. Alternatively you can tap it or massage the point instead of holding and breathing.

2.   Then press your right index finger tip into the side of your right hand thumb, like you did with your left hand. Repeat the Acupressure Desensitization Affirmation in your mind and take a deep breath. Alternatively you can tap it or stimulate this point in any other way you find the least conspicuous.

3.   Now press your left thumb into the side of your left index finger tip. Repeat your Acupressure Desensitization Affirmation and take a deep breath while thinking of your Acupressure Desensitization Affirmation. Alternatively, if you find taking a deep breath in public to conspicuous you can just massage the point with your finger or stimulate it in any other way we've listed above.

4.   Now release your left hand and press your right hand thumb on the side of your right hand index finger tip. And repeat the process again. Think of your Acupressure Desensitization Affirmation and either stimulate the point while breathing deeply and holding it or by massaging it or by pressing on it and releasing the pressure a few times.

5.   Now release your right hand and press your left hand thumb on the side of your left hand middle finger tip. Repeat your Acupressure Desensitization Affirmation in your mind and while doing this stimulate your acupressure point while thinking about it either by: breathing deeply while holding this acupressure point, massaging it by moving your thumb or by putting pressure on your thumb and releasing it interchangeably. The idea is to stimulate that acupoint, it doesn't matter how you do it.

6.   Now stop stimulating the acupoint on your right hand. And release your left hand and press your right hand thumb on the side of your right hand middle finger. Repeat your Accupressure Desensitization Affirmation in your mind and stimulate your acupoint.

7.   Release your right hand and press your left hand thumb on the side of your left ring finger tip. Repeat your Accupressure Desensitization Affirmation in your mind and stimulate your acupoint.

8.   Release your left hand and press your right hand thumb on the side of your right ring finger tip Repeat your Accupressure Desensitization Affirmation in your mind and stimulate your acupoint.

9.   Release your right hand and press your left hand thumb on the side of your left hand little finger Repeat your Accupressure Desensitization Affirmation in your mind and stimulate your acupoint

10.   Lastly, Release your left hand and press your right hand thumb into the side of your right hand little finger tip Repeat your Accupressure Desensitization Affirmation inr your mind and stimulate your acupoint

You can all of this while keeping your hands in your pocket. With this technique you'll be able to use AD even in public. You'll be able to calm down while anxious or angry. If your mind is too emotional to think straight you can also repeat this pocket AD sequence without thinking of anything special at all, you already have your problem ' in mind' when you're doing it in such a situation, and as such there's no need for you to repeat the Acupressure Desensitization Affirmation. Remember: The Acupressure Desensitization Affirmation's only purpose is to remind yourself of what you're working on during Acupressure desensitization. Nothing else. There's nothing special about it.

Repeat this until your Subjective Unit of Discomfort Reaches o. It's that simple.

You can use PAD whenever you have the urge to do porn. This is a simple method of combating relapses. You simply do PAD each time you think of porn or have an urge to do porn.

Exercise:

1: List the potential downsides of quitting porn:

Use them to create Acupressure Desensitization Affirmations and tap them out.

2: List the potential upsides of continuing using porn:

Use this setup phrase as a model;

"Even though <upside of porn> I still choose to quit porn"

'Even though I don't have to practice meditation to improve myself I still choose to quit porn', Then tap it out using Acupressure Desensitization to take the emotional charge away from these thoughts. Write down your experiences.

3: You can use AD to lower your craving when it gets too intense.

Next time you feel a porn craving do a tap session with the following setup phrase and AD affirmation:

"Even though I have this craving for porn, I deeply accept myself"

Or "Even though I have this urge to watch porn"

Or "Even though I'm craving porn..."

"Even though I feel anxious and want to watch porn to relax, I deeply accept myself"

ADA: This craving for porn

After the first round if there\'s still some craving left use this:

"Even though I still crave porn, I deeply and completely accept myself"

Repeat this until your craving will be lowered.

You'll learn a more advanced Version of this called **TAAP** in the relapse prevention module. But for now you can use this simplified version to manage your porn urges when they arise. Use the mindfulness skills you've learned so far to notice them. Write down your experience of using this technique if you managed to catch a craving and desensitize it.

4: THERE ARE SOME THOUGHTS THAT ARE COMMONLY IDENTIFIED IN ALL PORN ADDICTS

Just to be sure. Let's desensitize them now so that when they come up you'll have an easier time defusing from them.

Use these statements as setup phrases and do **AD** until you feel that they've been completely desensitized (SUD= 0)

Take note that the list of these statements is pretty long. Only choose the ones that you have an emotional response to. (SUD higher than 0) Repeat **AD** until you've completely desensitized the beliefs that have an associated negative charge.

1: Even if I never get over my porn problem, I deeply accept myself.

2: Even though I'm not worthy of having real partner, I deeply accept myself - This will take away the emotional charge from this belief, making it much easier for you to defuse from it

3: Even though it's not safe for me to quit porn, I accept myself.

4: Even though I know I'll feel deprived if I get over my porn problem, I deeply and completely accept myself.

5: Even though I'm afraid to let go of my porn addiction, I deeply and completely accept myself.

6: Even though I don't believe I can be free from porn, I deeply and completely accept myself.

7: Even though I don't trust myself to quit porn, I deeply and completely accept myself.

8: Even though I've never been successful/haven't been successful in the past, I accept myself.

9: Even though I'm afraid I will still be unhappy if I quit porn, I deeply accept myself.

10: Even though I can't give up my insecurity, I deeply and completely accept myself.

11: Even though I'm convinced I'll eventually relapse on porn, I deeply and completely accept myself.

12: Even though I don't deserve to be happy I deeply and completely accept myself.

13: Even though I'm afraid of success I deeply and completely accept myself.

14: Even though my sexuality is broken, I deeply and completely accept myself.

15: Even though I can't resist the urge to do porn, I deeply and completely accept myself.

5: Now let's do some compulsory tapings on something every porn addict should tap on

1: Even though I'm a porn addict, I deeply and completely accept myself.

2: Even though I crave porn after <put one of the triggers you've identified so far here, you can do this with every single one of your identified triggers>, I deeply and completely accept myself.

3: Even though I can't stay away from porn, I deeply and completely accept myself.

4: Even though I'm obsessed with porn, I deeply and completely accept myself.

5: Even though I think about porn all day long, I deeply and completely accept myself.

6: Even though thinking about porn makes me feel happy...

7: Even though I used porn as entertainment...

8: Even though I used porn as security...

9: Etc.

6: DESENSITIZE YOUR SEXUAL FANTASIES

This technique can also be used to desensitize any form of compulsive sexual fantasy you might have. For example I couldn't stop thinking about morbidly obese women. Whenever I had a period of free time I would think about them. No matter how hard I tried I couldn't defuse from that thought, because it would continue haunting me every second of my life. Acupressure desensitization allowed me to lower the power of that thought and become free from it.

'Even though I can't stop thinking about < the intrusive thought you have>, I deeply and completely accept myself'

'Even though I think about< your obsessive thought>, I deeply and completely accept myself'

7: LET'S DESENSITIZE YOUR TRIGGERS

Do you remember when we asked you to list your triggers? I want to use the story technique to desensitize every single trigger you've written down so far. Simply tell a story about it and start tapping and apply AD when you notice a craving.

For example I would tell this story: I'm seeing a morbidly obese girl on the street. I see her stomach hanging from her blouse; it's obvious that her clothes are too tight for her because of her size. I get an erection. I can't stop thinking about it <at this point of the story I feel a craving for pornography>

The setup phrase here would be: Even though I feel a craving for porn each time I see a fat girl, I accept myself.

The AD affirmation would be: Craving for porn each time I see a fat girl.

Write down all of the statements you've tapped out in your journal.

8: Let's desensitize the times you're most prone to porn

Do you remember when we asked you to write down the times you feel the most prone to do porn? And your triggers? Well now it's the time to tap on all of them.

Here are some examples to help you get started:

Even though I feel the urge to do porn in the morning...

Even though I watch porn when I'm alone...

Even though I watch porn during work...

9: Now ask yourself: How do you feel about yourself as a porn addict?

Negative beliefs about yourself fuel your porn addiction. By taking away their emotional charge through AD we're taking away their power, making it much easier for you to defuse from them when they appear in your mind.

"Even though I'm ashamed of myself for being a porn addict..."

"Even though I'm ashamed that <insert your weird sexual prefer-ence>" For example: "Even though I'm ashamed that I'm attracted to women gaining weight, I choose to accept myself."

10: IMAGINE THAT ALL PORN IN THE WORLD WAS DESTROYED AND IT WAS BANNED BY THE DEATH PENALTY. HOW WOULD YOU FEEL?

You might want to tell a story/write out to identify anything with emotional salience. Here are some suggestions:

'Even though I feel angry when I am deprived...'

'Even though I feel panicky when I can't watch porn when I want...'

'Even though I feel afraid when I don't have free access to porn..'

If you can't find out anything unique. Tap out these. Write down everything you've tapped out.

11: SOMETIMES OUR ADDICTIVE URGES ARE FUELED BY OUR PAST. WHAT EVENTS FROM THE PAST MAKE YOU FEEL ANXIOUS/GUILTY/ASHAMED?

Use The Tell a Story technique you've learned in this lesson to de-sensitize them using AD. Try doing this on any other past events that might be fueling your porn addiction.

For example here are some of my past events that contributed to my porn addiction:

'Even though I was bullied by skinny chicks at school and wanted to take revenge on them by forcibly fattening them up, I deeply and completely accept myself'

'Even though when I was a kid I felt that I could only win friends by giving porn away, I forgive myself and accept myself.'

Write down everything you desensitized in this exercise. Write down your setup phrases, and AD affirmations, and whether or not you were successful at desensitizing them. Write down the before and after ratings.

12: WHAT PAST MEMORIES AND THOUGHTS OR EMOTIONS ARE YOU NUMBING THROUGH PORN USE?

List them and desensitize them using AD. That will make it much easier for you to be present with them when they come up:

Here are mine:

'Even though I feel that I'll never achieve anything in my life, I deeply and completely accept myself'

'Even though I feel that I'm ugly and stupid and unlovable, I forgive myself and choose to accept myself as I am'

'Even though I feel overwhelmed with life and want to escape, I forgive myself and accept myself'

13: THINK OF THE FIRST TIME YOU'VE USED PORN. DESENSITIZE IT USING AD

That memory will then stop fueling your current addiction. Here's an example:

'Even though I never before felt as good as when I did porn for the first time, I choose to quit porn and I forgive myself.'

14: REMEMBER WHEN YOU WROTE ALL THE POTENTIAL TRIGGERS IN YOUR JOURNAL. IMAGINE YOU ARE EXPOSED TO THEM IN THE FUTURE AND DESENSITIZE THEM USING AD

Write a story about them and desensitize every part of the story that has any craving or any other emotional charge. Here are some examples set up phrases to give you an idea:

'Even though I'll know I'll relapse when I'll see a fat girl on the street, I deeply and completely accept myself'

'Even though I know I'll relapse after hearing or reading about feederism, I forgive myself and choose not to do that'

Write down all of the setup phrases and AD affirmation you've used in your journal.

15: THINK OF ANY OTHER NEGATIVE CONSEQUENCES THAT MIGHT OCCUR IF YOU QUIT PORN FOREVER. LIST THEM AND DESENSITIZE THEM USING AD

Write out all of them in your journal. Here's an example:

'Even though I don't know what I'll do with the freed up time once I quit porn, I deeply and completely accept myself.'

16: PICTURE YOURSELF AS BEING PORN FREE. DESCRIBE IT WITH A STORY. WHAT FEELINGS OR THOUGHTS ARISE IN YOUR MIND WHEN YOU DO THIS? TREAT ALL THE NEGATIVE ONES WITH AD.

For example:

'Even though I don't believe I could really be porn free...'

'Even though I don't identify with being porn free...'

'Even though I'm afraid I'll fail at quitting...'

'Even though my online friends pressure me to watch porn again...' (This is relevant if you were either in the BDSM or furry community in the past)

Write down all the setup phrases and AD affirmations you've used in the past.

17: Now I want you to imagine having withdrawal symptoms. Tap it out using ADD

Here are some example setup phrases to stimulate your imagination:

'Even though I fear having nightmares when I quit...'

'Even though I'm afraid of physical withdrawal...'

'Even though I know I might be irritable in the beginning of quitting porn...'

'Even though I can't imagine living without porn...'

Write down everything you desensitized in this exercise. Write down your setup phrases, and AD affirmations, and whether or not you were successful at desensitizing them. Write down the before and after ratings.

18: Are there any feelings of loss related to quitting porn? List them out and desensitize them using AD

Examples:

'Even though I miss my porn...'

'Even though I feel I have lost a friend...'
'Even though I feel sad about quitting porn...'

Write down everything you desensitized in this exercise. Write down your setup phrases, and **AD** affirmations, and whether or not you were successful at desensitizing them. Write down the before and after ratings.

19: WHAT OTHER LOSSES HAVE BEEN TRIGGERED BY QUITTING PORN? APPLY AD TO EACH ONE

'Even though I keep thinking about the loss of my father/mother/friend...'
'Even though I feel sadness about my family...'

20: DO YOU HAVE ANY ANXIETY ABOUT QUITTING PORN AND BEING WITHOUT PORN FOR THE REST OF YOUR LIFE? LIST IT OUT AND TAP IT OUT USING AD

'Even though I feel anxious being porn free...'
'Even though I don't believe in myself'
'Even though I'm afraid to succeed fail...'
'Even though I don't know what to do with my time if I don't use porn...'
'Even though I'm the only man I know who doesn't use porn now...'

Write down everything you desensitized in this exercise. Write down your setup phrases, and **AD** affirmations, and whether or not you were successful at desensitizing them. Write down the before and after ratings.

21: HOW DO YOU FEEL AFTER YOU SEE OR HEAR ABOUT PORN?

Use The Tell a Story technique to describe how you feel after you see porn or hear about porn. Tap out anything that comes up that has any emotional charge. Write down all of the statements you've tapped out below

Here are some examples:

'Even though I feel I absolutely must masturbate after I see porn..."

'Even though I have the compulsion to masturbate even after reading about porn..."

You can also be more specific. Here\'s my example:

'Even though I want to masturbate each time I see an overweight woman...'

Remember you can't do too much AD. Do as much of it as you can. Write down your affirmations, your SUDS etc.

22: USE PAD COVERTLY

Try using Pad on a problem either outside or somewhere else with people. Practice doing it covertly. Just put your hands in your pocket and stimulate your acupoints. Write down your experiences. Were you able to successfully do that?

[12]

How To Move From A Porn-Driven Life To A Purpose Driven Life

LET ME NOW GIVE YOU the official definition of values in Acceptance and Commitment Therapy (Harris, 2009).

"Values are freely chosen ways you understand your place in the world; they are patterns of behavior that evolve over time based on your actions, and you feel satisfaction mainly by doing these actions for their own sake, not for any outside incentive or rewards."

Values are our heart's deepest desires for the way we want to interact with the world, other people, and ourselves. They're what we want to stand for in life, how we want to behave, what sort of person we want to be, what sort of strengths and qualities we want to develop.

I know the technical jargon might be confusing but allow me to dissect this definition so that everyone can understand it:
LET'S NOW DISSECT THIS DEFINITION:

Values are freely chosen. Your values are Your Own. They are not society's values or your parents' values. We won't tell you what you should value and we suggest that you won't allow anyone else to tell you that either. During my new age days, I allowed 'authorities' to tell me what I should value or not, and that was one of the worst decisions of my life.

You're the one who has to choose your own values in life.

But at the same time, just because you're the one choosing your value doesn't mean that you'll always be a perfect example of them. You might choose that you value your relationship with your children very highly. Does this mean you'll always be the perfect parent? There will be times when you'll do things that are incompatible with your idea of what it means to be a good parent. Your basic choice to make this area of your life a priority is what constitutes your values.

VALUES DESCRIBE YOUR UNDERSTANDING OF YOUR PLACE IN THE WORLD

When we're talking about values, we're going to mean those ways in which you've decided to relate yourself to the role you will play in the world- as a member of a community or family, as an artist, as a writer, as a teacher and so forth.

VALUES ARE PATTERNS OF BEHAVIOR

Values are not individual acts. You're not a good husband just because you once buy flowers for your wife. In this case, a value would be a pattern of acts that show consideration, thoughtfulness and kindness. Giving flowers might be part of the pattern, but it's only a small part of it. A value pattern is something that will make someone stand at your graveside and say: "he was a loving husband". Values are something you ARE, they are not one-shot acts that you do and then forget. They are also not goals that you achieve and are done with. They are something you practice all of your life.

VALUE AREN'T STATIC. THEY ARE DYNAMIC AND DEVELOP BASED ON YOUR ACTIONS

For example, the value of 'being a good husband' changes over time. Different things make a 'good husband' at age 20 and at age 50. Our patterns of living change, even though the central value remains the same. Some people might understand values as some kind of code of conduct, but in our understanding values evolve over time as a result of many, many actions you might take in the service of patterns of living you care about.

At the same time we don't really 'clarify' or 'discover' our values. We construct it over time as we engage in a pattern of action that starts to look like a value. Once you decide what you want your life to be about, only your efforts over time can really work out for you what this actually means.

VALUES ARE INTRINSICALLY REWARDING

A value is something that one doesn't do to 'get something,' it's something you find reward in for its own sake. The only reason to be a good father is the reward of being a good father. Values are something that are intrinsically rewarding and don't need an outside reward to be rewarding.

At some point in your life, you might find that nothing is rewarding. I hope that the exercises in this course will help you find at least one value in your life.

IT'S IMPORTANT TO NOTE THAT VALUES ARE NOT FEELINGS

If someone bases action on the absence or presence of emotions, he cannot lead a value driven life. Emotional obstacles will always arise, and they'll ask you "will you have me?" If you answer 'no' the journey will stop. We need to learn to value even when we don't feel like it, to love even when we feel angry, to care even when we feel despair.

VALUES ARE CHOICES

They don't need to be explained, justified, or in any way guided by our verbal evaluations and judgments. A value is not a decision. Let me explain the difference. A decision is a selection among alternative courses of action made for a reason; reasons are collections of pros and cons. When you make a decision that decision is justified, explained and guided by reasons. For example, you might invest in apple stock because you think that that company will grow in value, and because it has a strong record of growth. These are reasons that justify and explain the purchase of the stock. Choices are something else.

VALUES ARE NOT GOALS

Values are the directions we're going. They are a like a compass for life. A compass gives you direction and keeps you on track when you're traveling; your values do the same for the journey of life. We use them to choose the direction in which we want to move and to keep us on track as we go. So when you act on a value, it's like heading west. No matter how far west you travel, you never get there; there's always further you can go. They are not a goal to cross off a list. They are our principles that guide every choice we've made in our life. For example, if you want to be a good and loving partner, that's a value. Once you're no longer a loving partner, you're no longer practicing that value. On the other hand, marriage is a goal. It can be accomplished and crossed off your to do list. Once you're married, you're married even if you start treating your partner badly. Having a job is a goal, but being good at one's job is a value. It's an ongoing process. On the other hand, goals are like the things you try to achieve on your journey of life; they're like the sights you want to see or the mountains you want to climb while you keep on traveling west.

VALUES NEVER NEED TO BE JUSTIFIED

Goals need explanation and reasons for their experience. On the other hand, values never need to be justified. They are your choices and as such you don't need to explain or justify them to anyone.

VALUES ARE HERE AND NOW; GOALS ARE IN THE FUTURE

As you'll learn in future lessons, goals are something that you plan. They are something that you structure your daily activities around. In contrast, values are something you practice moment by moment. Once you become more conscious of your behavior through mindfulness, you'll notice that you're consciously making choices on how to behave every moment of your life. Once your values will be clear to you, you'll be able to make the right choices. This will allow you to choose to not to use porn when the urge porn appears in your mind, because you'll have something better to do than that.

VALUES OFTEN NEED TO BE PRIORITIZED

Life is not perfect. Sometimes you'll have to choose one value over another. That's why in a lesson that follows after the next lesson you'll learn to how to effectively prioritize your values, so you'll know exactly how to behave in every moment of your life.

VALUES ARE BEST HELD LIGHTLY

The mind can sometimes transform even values into a destructive force. It does so when it turns the statement "I choose to be a good parent" into the statement "I must be a good parent".
Rational Emotive Behavioral Therapy and Cognitive Behavioral Therapy have known for decades that thought patterns including

'musts' are the most self-destructive. As you know after you went through the previous module. I just want you to keep in mind that when you think of your values it's better to think of them in terms of "I choose to be a good partner" rather than "I must be a good partner."

SUCCESS IS LIVING BY YOUR VALUES

With this definition you can be successful right now even though your goals maybe a long way off. Let me now tell you a story about the importance of prioritizing your values:

A professor stood before his class with a large empty jar over his table. He filled the empty jar with Ping-Pong balls and asked the students if the jar was full. They agreed that it was. Then the professor picked up a container of small rocks and poured them into the jar so they filled the spaces between the Ping-Pong balls. Again, he asked the students if the jar was full. They agreed it was. Next, the professor picked up a bag of sand and poured it into the jar, filling the spaces between the small stones. He asked once more if the jar was full. The students responded with a unanimous yes. The professor then said, "This jar represents your life. The Ping-Pong balls are the important things -Your family, your kids, your physical health, your friendships, and your passions- things that if everything else was lost and only they remained, your life would still be full. The small rocks are the other things that matter, like your career, your home, and your car. The sand is everything else -the little stuff. If you put the sand in the jar first, you won't be able to fit all of the little rocks, let alone the Ping-Pong balls. The same goes for life. If you spend all of your time and energy on the little stuff, you won't have space for the things that are most vital to you. Make time for the things that are crucial to a meaningful life. Play with your kids. Take time to see your doctor. Go on a date with your spouse or partner. Go on vacation. There will always be time to do the chores and change the light bulbs. Prioritize the Ping-Pong balls first, the things that really matter. The rest is just sand."

IDENTIFYING YOUR VALUES IS LIKE CREATING A SOLID FOUNDATION FOR YOUR HOME

Imagine remodeling your home. You're excited to choose attractive new tiles and modern appliances and to paint the walls in exciting new colors. Your budget is set, and you have everything all planned out, but then you find out that there's a major crack in the foundation of your home. Trying to figure out how to live your life (how to solve this problem, how to make this choice, and so on) before you decide who you really want to be and what you want to stand for would be like going forward with your remodel without fixing the foundation. If you hang pretty drapes and lay cozy carpets but your foundation is broken, your house will ultimately start to lean or cave in. You need to spend some extra time and money now to repair the foundation properly, and this may mean you can't immediately afford the attractive tile and modern appliances. However, at the end of the day, you'll have a solid home and less to worry about.

Living in alignment with your values doesn't guarantee that everything you want will occur or that you'll necessarily feel comfortable. But you will know that you're on the right track, and you'll be living a fuller, richer, more meaningful life that's congruent with the person you want to be. Living a valued life means that even when things don't go perfectly, not only will you still be standing; you'll maintain the integrity of the building.

Once you define your values you'll be able to choose the direction of your life intentionally and on purpose moment to moment. Once you find-out your life's purpose (your values) you'll be able to let go of a preoccupation with immediate gratification and immediate outcomes and instead life a value-driven life in the moment, even when the moment itself is unpleasant. You have no real control on whether or not you'll achieve your goals. But you can choose to act in a valued direction every moment of your life.

Your values will ultimately be the main thing that will help you overcome your porn addiction. Whenever you're addicted self says: "Why am I doing this? Why I am I going through all of this effort to quit porn", you can say: "Because it's something that matters to me. Because I choose this life."

Coming up next I'm giving you to do the longest succession of exercises we've done yet. But don't worry; you're allowed more than one day to put them in practice.

EXERCISE

Let's now look at your values in the main life domains, starting with; Relationships:

• What sort of brother/sister, son/daughter, uncle/aunt do you want to be?

• What sort of relationships would you like to build?

• How would you interact with others if you were the ideal you in these relationships?

• What sort of partner would you like to be in an intimate relationship?

• What personal qualities would you like to develop?

• What sort of relationship would you like to build?

• How would you interact with your partner if you were the 'ideal you' in this relationship?

Parenting:

• What sort of parent would you like to be?

• What sort of qualities would you like to have?

- What sort of relationships would you like to build with your children?
- How would you behave if you were the 'ideal you'?

Friendships/Social life:

- What sort of qualities would you like to bring to your friendships?
- If you could be the best friend possible, how would you behave towards your friends?
- What sort of friendships would you like to build?

Career/Employment:

- What do you value in your work?
- What would make it more meaningful?
- What kind of worker would you like to be?
- If you were living up to your own ideal standards, what personal qualities would you like to bring to your work?
- What sort of work relations would you like to build?
- How do you want to be towards your clients, customers, colleagues, employees, fellow workers?
- What personal qualities do you want to bring to your work?
- What skills do you want to develop?

Education/Personal growth and development:

- What do you value about learning, education, training, or personal growth?
- What knowledge would you like to gain?
- What new skills would you like to learn?
- What further education appeals to you?
- What sort of student would you like to be?
- What personal qualities would you like to apply?

Recreation/Fun/Leisure:

• What sorts of hobbies, sports, or leisure activities do you enjoy?

• How do you relax and unwind?

• How do you have fun?

• What sorts of activities would you like to do?

• Referring to how you play, relax, stimulate, or enjoy yourself; your hobbies or other activities for rest, recreation, fun and creativity, how would the ideal you spend his/her free time?

Spirituality:

• Whatever spirituality means to you is fine. It may be as simple as communing with nature, or as formal as participation in an organized religious group. What is important to you in this area of life?

Citizenship/Environment/Community life:

• How would you like to contribute to your community or environment, e.g. through volunteering, or recycling, or supporting a group/charity/ political party?

• What sort of environments would you like to create at home, and at work? What environments would you like to spend more time in?

Health/Physical well-being:

• What are your values related to maintaining your physical well-being?

• How do you want to look after your health, with regard to sleep, diet, exercise, smoking, alcohol, etc?

• Why is this important?

EXERCISE

I would ask you to try on at least one value (you can do it with more).

You'll be required to write about your experiences with a given value in your journal. This will give you a direct experiential proof of whether or not a value is right for you.

1.   **Choose a value:** Choose a valued direction that you're willing to try on for at least a week. This should be a value that you can enact and that you care about. This isn't a time to try to change others or manipulate them into changing.

2.   **Notice reactions:** Notice anything that comes up about whether or not this is a "good" value, or whether you really care about this value. Just notice all thoughts for what they are. Remember that your mind's job is to create thoughts. Let your mind do that while you continue with the exercise.

3.   **Make a list:** Take a moment to list a few behaviors that are related to the chosen value.

4.   **Choose a behavior:** From this list, choose a behavior or set of behaviors that you can commit to doing between now and the next session or the next few sessions.

5.   **Notice judgments:** Notice anything that comes up about whether or not that's a good behavior, whether you'll enjoy it, or whether you can actually do the action you're committing to.

6.   **Make a plan:** Write down how you'll go about enacting this value in the very near future (today, tomorrow, this weekend, and so on). Consider anything you'll need to plan or get in order, such as calling someone, cleaning the house, or making an appointment. Choose when to do that--the sooner, the better.

7.   **Just behave:** Even if this value involves other people, don't tell them what you're doing. See what you can notice if you just enact this value without telling others about the experiment you're doing.

8.   **Commit:** Commit to following your plan every day. Notice anything that shows up as you do so.

9.　　　**Keep a daily diary of your reactions:** Things to look for and record in your diary include other people's reactions to you; any thoughts, feelings, or bodily sensations that occur before, during, or after the behavior; and how you feel doing your chosen action for the second (or fifth, or tenth, or hundredth) time. Watch for evaluations that indicate whether this activity, value, or valued direction was "good" or "bad" or judgments about others or yourself in relation to living this value. Gently thank your mind for those thoughts and see if you can choose not to buy into the judgments your mind makes about the activity.

10.　　　**Reflect.**

EXERCISE FILL OUT THE VALUE QUESTIONNAIRE

Domain	Current importance	Overall importance	Possibility of action	Satisfied/Concerned with level of action	Total
Family					
Intimate relationships					
Parenting					
Friends and social life					
Work					
Education and training					
Recreation and fun					
The environment					
Spirituality					
Community life					
Physical care					
Creativity					

Remember. You can make up/create any value you'd like, as long as it is a value. Feel free to draw the table on your journal so you can use as much space as you need.

FINDING VALUES IN UNENJOYABLE ACTIVITIES

The next exercise will teach you how to find something valuable in unenjoyable activities

There are many things we do that we don't particularly enjoy. Sometimes we do things that aren't enjoyable in the moment because they're linked to something we care about. For example, a spouse may not particularly enjoy taking out the trash, but they do it anyway because of their values in regard to being a good partner.

This worksheet can help you to see if there's anything you care about inside some unenjoyable activities. There are no right answers here; this worksheet is simply designed to help you see if there is something of value to you in an unenjoyable activity; There may or may not be.

On your journal write down an unenjoyable activity now, and then consider the possible reasons why you do this activity (for example, someone or something that is important to you in some way would be negatively affected if you didn't do it). Write these reasons down. In your journal, record the thoughts, feelings, and bodily sensations you notice when you do this activity.

Is there a value inside even one of your reasons for doing this behavior? If so, describe it now:

If yes, list three ways you can choose to do to live this value this week. You can include the original behavior above if you wish. In the spaces to the left, record your willingness to do each using a scale of 0 to 10, in which 0 indicates not at all willing and 10 indicates very willing:

You might find that even at this point you might have a hard time with coming up with values, and instead you come up with a lot of goals such as "I would like to be wealthy" or "I would like to have fame " or "I want to have a good job" or "I want to have a very fit body". I would like you to invite you to an exercise designed to identify the value hidden within a goal.

Ask yourself these questions:

- If this goal was achieved, what would you do differently?
- If this goal was achieved, how would you act differently?
- If this goal was achieved, how would you behave differently in your relationships, work life, social life, and family life and so on?
- If this goal was achieved, what personal qualities or strengths would it demonstrate?
- If this goal was achieved, what would it show that you stand for?
- If this goal was achieved, what would it enable you to do that is meaningful and that matters in the big picture?

EXERCISE

THINK ABOUT YOUR HEROES. CONSIDER PEOPLE WHO HAVE PLAYED A DIRECT ROLE IN YOUR LIFE: FAMILY MEMBERS, FRIENDS, TEACHERS, COACHES, TEAMMATES, AND SO ON. NOW THINK ABOUT PEOPLE WHO HAVE INSPIRED YOU INDIRECTLY: AUTHORS, ARTISTS, CELEBRITIES, OR EVEN FICTIONAL CHARACTERS. WHO WOULD YOU LIKE TO BE LIKE THE MOST? PICK ONE PERSON YOU REALLY ADMIRE.

Now think about all the qualities you really admire in this person -Not the person's circumstances, but personal qualities- and write them down. Once you've done this, I'd like you to look this over and think about how these might translate into your own personal values. Now on your journal, write down as follows and answer the following questions:

- What's the name of your hero?
- What values that this person embodies do you admire?
- How can you move toward being more like your hero?
- What Actions you can take to start moving in the direction of being more like your hero?
- What skills and/or exercises you might use to handle obstacles (e.g., thoughts, feelings, urges, memories) that might get in the way toward being more like your hero?
- What can you do to move forward? (Like your hero would)

You can do this for another hero since most people admire more than one person. Simply answer the same questions from above with your newly picked hero.

Your Personal Job Ad

At some point in our life's we've seen a job advertisement, be it on TV, Newspapers, internet, you name it. The trick to get the job is to match the job description given to us. But what would happen if you described yourself as an organization? Imagine that there's a new jobs section in the newspaper, but instead of having organizations advertising specific jobs, it contains information about people offering themselves, and employers check if they can provide a role that meets the candidate's requirements. Write your personal job ad, advertising to the world the kind of person you are and what you care about, but don't specify a particular job or profession. Make sure that your ad includes the following:

- Your name and maybe a personal motto
- Personal qualities, such as generous, impatient, or introverted
- Talents or skills, such as playing the trombone or designing spreadsheets
- Values, such as wanting to make a difference

- Ambitions, such as "I want to run my own business" or "I want to be paid well enough to take vacations twice a year"
- Anything else you wish for in your ideal job, such as "I want a job where I can be an expert (Computers, can use my Spanish, can travel, and so on)"
- Jobs that need not apply, such as "I don't want a job that requires travel"
- One thing you cannot compromise on, such as "I won't take a job where I can't be outdoors"

Here's an example:

Name and motto: Bob Bowman. The best in me brings out the best in others.

Personal qualities: Open, curious, generous, compassionate, anxious, ambitious, courageous, bright, determined.

Talents: Social intelligence, psychology and counseling, sports, creativity,

Values: Meaning, freedom, status, courage, integrity

Ambitions: I want to build something. I want to make a difference to other people. I want to build a movement that changes the way people see work. I want to use psychology to help people cope with their suffering.

Anything else you wish for in your ideal job: I want to be an expert in something and to pass this expertise on. I want to build effective tools that help people move forward and to make these accessible for free. I want to be very well paid, but want this to reflect my value to others. I want to write brilliant books that aren't afraid to challenge convention. I want to travel a bit. I want to live in the United States one day. I want to have a family and dedicate time to them. I want to work with brilliant, like-minded people.

Jobs that need not apply: Anything to do with bureaucracy. Selling things that people don't need. Anything that has no evidence to support it. Anything that relies on drinking.

One thing you cannot compromise on: My values.

EXERCISE

Let's now slowly explore different areas of your life to see if you can find something you value in them. As you do this exercise, there might be some resistance. If resistances occurs, I would like you to ask yourself: "Could I open myself up to this experience?" or simply apply the mindful question method. Whichever you'll find easier. Before your start this exercise I would like you to ask yourself: "Could I let go of all condemnation for now?"

If the answer is No, do the exercise later when the answer is Yes. You can always condemn yourself later. There'll be plenty of time for that, but for now I want you to make this a time of no-self condemnation.

Below you'll find a list of 12 areas of your life:

- **Relationships**
- **Work**
- **Friends**
- **Education and learning**
- **Recreation and fun**
- **Spirituality**
- **Community life**
- **Physical care, exercise, sleep, nutrition**
- **Art, music, literature and beauty.**
- **Parenting**

I would like you to pick 3 areas of your life to reflect on. Become aware of it and gently allow yourself to become aware of ways you've been absent, of times when you could have been present but weren't.

It is fine if examples don't come up. There are no right or wrong answers, and this exercise is not about doing anything. Its purpose is for you to learn how to notice and gently shift your attention and about learning how to be present and mindful. There's nothing to accomplish here other than to notice and ponder.

Just open yourself up to your experience. If something flows in, let it. If something spills out, that's also perfectly okay.

If while doing the exercise you might find yourself caught in worry or rumination. Close your eyes ask yourself: "Can I just open up to this experience?' And then notice the sensation of your breath. Then gently take your attention back to the inventory.

I want you to know that this is **NOT** an exercise in determining 'what's wrong with you'. Thoughts like that WILL show up in this exercise, and we want you to practice defusion, presence and willingness with them, as this is what this exercise is truly aimed to do: To train your mindfulness muscle. The purpose of this exercise is to start learning to apply mindfulness skills in uncomfortable situations. In this exercise you'll practice pausing, and coming to presence when your mind produces uncomfortable feelings.

To make this exercise easier I will show you how hiding, fighting and some other activities of your mind you'll defuse from will look like:

Hiding: "I don't need to do this."

Running: "I'll do this later."

Fighting: "**WHY DO I NEED TO DO THIS?** It seems uncomfortable and unpleasant. What does this have to do with quitting my porn addiction anyway? You can't make me do this!"

All of these thoughts will be in fact true. (Except the part that says that this doesn't have anything to do with your porn addiction. It has everything to do with managing your addiction. By becoming more mindful and present you'll be able to manage your urges far more effectively)

At this point in the value construction process I want you to let go off trying to 'solve anything' we're just non-judgmentally observing your life. Goal setting, planning, and 'problem-solving' will come later. At this point we're only observing and witnessing. That's why I would like you to defuse any thoughts about what's possible or impossible. Whenever you'll find your mind using words like 'can't', 'should', 'shouldn't', 'possible', 'impossible', I want you to just take a few breaths and get back into the present moment.

Answer these questions:

- Deep down inside, what is important to you?
- What do you want your life to stand for?
- What sort of qualities do you want to cultivate as a person?
- How do you want to be in your relationships with others?
- If you could wave a magic wand so that all of your problematic thoughts and feelings no longer had an impact on you, what would you start doing, or do more of?
- What would you stop doing, or do less of?
- Do you ever feel a sense of purpose, meaning, vitality, or fulfillment -Even for just a moment? Doing what? What, when, where, how, and with whom?
- If, in the process of dealing with your porn addiction, you could develop some personal strength, qualities or abilities that would help you in some way to become a "better person", to "grow as a human being," or "make a difference in the lives of others," what might those strengths, qualities, or abilities be?
- What are you doing in your life right now that is inconsistent with the person, deep in your heart, that you truly want to be? What would you like to do differently?

- If the work we do here on your porn addiction could have a positive impact on the most important relationships in your life, which relationships would improve? And how? How would you like to be in those relationships if you could be the ideal you?
- What do you want to stand for in the face of your porn addiction?
- If at some point in the future you were to look back at the way you handled this situation now, then what would you like to say about the way you handled it?
- What would you like to say about how you grew or developed as a result of it?

TRAPS THAT KEEP YOU FROM LIVING A VALUE-LED LIFE

I would like to discuss three traps that might keep you from living a valued existence.

Trap One: Experiential avoidance
Many people think that they need to feel good in order to do well. Some people might choose "I value feeling good so that I might be x" The truth is that you can be x no matter what you feel. All you need is cognitive defusion.

Trap 2: Keeping up appearances
Many people do things just to please others and not because they actually value them. We're conditioned to please our elders and the people around us and to do things because we want people to praise us. Many people find it hard to create their own values as opposed to their parents values. The professional term for this is pliancy.

Trap 3 Living for the rewards

As I mentioned in the previous lessons, values are something that are rewarding on their own merit. I want you to ask you a few questions now that might show some values that you might have that are independent of any conventional rewards such as money and fame. We also have to remember balance while pursuing our values. This metaphor will illustrate that:

Imagine that you're an aerospace engineer and you're sitting at a control panel watching an aircraft flight on a screen in front of you. Your job is to adjust the dials that control the weight, lift, drag, and thrust of the aircraft in order to keep it flying effectively. All of these elements are equally important, and if you don't make the needed adjustments, the plane won't be able to fly effectively. You have to find the right balance for the smoothest flight. Now, although you have control over these adjustments, other factors remain out of your control. For example, you didn't design or build the aircraft. You can't control the weather. If the engine fails, this isn't your fault. But if you get hooked by worries about the factors that are out of your control, it may impact your adjustment of the weight, lift, drag, and thrust, and this may negatively impact your flight. The important thing here is to focus on the factors you can control and keep them in balance for the smoothest flight. If the weather happens to get rough or an engine does fail, your job is to do what you need to do to keep the plane in the air.

Some of you might not have the words to adequately express your values, so here's a list of words that may help you generate ideas about your values. Note that some of these words, like Calm, Patience, and Courage, may refer to internal experiences. In these cases, the value may be to <u>ACT</u> calmly or with patience or courage, even if you don't feel this way. The value should <u>not</u> be to achieve an internal feeling state.

-Adventure

-Attentiveness
-Balance
-Beauty
-Belonging
-Calm
-Caring
-Citizenship
-Comfort
-Communication
-Compassion
-Connectedness
-Conservation
-Courage
-Creativity
-Curiosity
-Detachment
-Discipline
-Diversity
-Effort
-Equality
-Excitement
-Expansiveness
-Experience
-Faith
-Fitness
-Flow
-Forgiveness
-Freedom
-Fun
-Health
-Honor
-Humor

-Imagination
-Independence
-Integrity
-Intelligence
-Interdependence
-Intimacy
-Intuition
-Justice
-Kindness
-Leadership
-Learning
-Love
-Loyalty
-Magic
-Meaning
-Nesting
-Nurturance
-Openness
-Order
-Organization
-Patience
-Peace
-Perseverance
-Play
-Power
-Productivity
-Reliability
-Respect
-Reverence
-Rhythm
-Risk
-Security

-Self-expression

-Self-sufficiency

-Sensuality

-Serenity

-Simplicity

-Spirituality

-Spontaneity

-Stability

-Stewardship

-Strength

-Structure

-Sustainability

-Thoughtfulness

-Tolerance

-Transcendence

-Understanding-

-Warmth

-Wisdom

-Wit

-Wonder

MY VALUED LIFE EPITAPH

Imagine that you could live your life without being controlled by your negative thoughts and emotion. As you connect with this imagine that you're looking at the headstone on your grave. What epitaph (words describing your life) would you like to see on your headstone? Think of a phrase or a series of brief statements that would capture the essence of the life you want to lead. What is it you want to be remembered for? If you could train your mindfulness skills and lived your life without being controlled by thoughts and emotions what would you be doing with your time and energy?

Write the answer to this question on your journal. Think big. There are no limits. If you're going to be thinking anything, you might as well think big.

I just want to note that this isn't a hypothetical exercise. Your values and whether or not you'll uphold your commitment to stand by those values will determine what you'll be remembered for.

The reason why so far in the NoPorn plan we focused more on all-round self-development than directly quitting your porn addiction is because we know that to truly quit porn addiction you need a set of well-developed values. If you don't, your tombstone might read like this:

Here lies John: He spent most of his life struggling with pornography.

Or if you followed our exercises through it could read like this:

Here lies John: He managed his porn addiction and lived a happy, fullfilling life.

Instead we want your tombstone to have something on it that you'd be proud of. Write the epitaph of the you you want to be right now on your journal.

COMMITMENT STARTS A NEW PATH IN LIFE

The work that we're doing here is like walking across a wild hillside. This work is brand new, so there's no path to walk on. Every step may be effortful, and deliberate effort is needed to keep taking steps. Then you look over to your right and see a well-worn path. It looks like it would be so much easier to walk on that path than to keep persisting on this unmarked route across the tall, overgrown grass.

The thing is, you know exactly where that well-worn path goes because you've walked it so many times before. Where does that path lead in your life?

We're walking together across new territory, and sometimes it's not so easy. Then you see that old, familiar path...

What have you learned from our work together that could be useful to you in those moments when you notice that you're being pulled onto that old familiar path?

What will it take for this new path to eventually become well-worn and easier to walk on?

Let's spend a moment noticing and contacting the direction this new path is traveling. Where does this new path lead? What are some of the things we could see along this new path?

In your journal I want you to write down one of the values you've identified in the previous lesson and then I want you to write a few actions (As many as you see fitting) that you could take that are consistent with that value. Here is a small Example:

My value is: Being a good husband
1 Taking out the trash
2 Remembering her birthday
3 buying flowers for her every now and then

LEARN HOW TO COMMIT IN THE PRESENT TO BE THE BEST YOU CAN BE

Commitment is all about what you do in the present. "Will I masturbate in the future?" We don't know. Don't ask yourself this question. Ask yourself "Will I masturbate now?" Right now? No. What about now? Renew this commitment again and again, moment by moment.

Try to defuse from all rumination about whether or not the commitment is right for you. Once you've committed to it, you've made the choice. You can change your choice later on of course. But I want you to do 'on paper' while you're working or doing something 'in the real world' I always want you to assume that all of your values are as you picked them. You change your values on paper, in your journal. Just like how you picked your journal. This will make your values seem more serious to you. If you commit to act in the preset moment in ways that are consistent with your values, you'll be free from porn. It's as simple as that.

Since we changed our definition of success, we're less concerned with achieving our goals than with acting in accordance to our values moment by moment. Although we will discuss how to set goals and manage time in a way that's in alignment with Acceptance and Commitment therapy.

The outcomes of our commitments aren't something we have much control over in real life, but we can always commit to doing something in the moment that will get us a little closer to something that matters to us. If we fail to uphold our values in one moment, we'll find ourselves in a new moment where can turn back toward our values. This turning back is at the heart of successful recovery.

We choose our values and we transform them into deeds with commitment.

"I will be a good father to my child."

"I will be kind."

"I will be a good worker."

"I will excel in my profession".

We make promises about the future, and we fail. The most loving parent might be a bastard sometimes, and the most productive worker might not do the best job. Upholding the values is less about achievement and more about commitment.

We always stray from our values and redirect ourselves back to them. The Breathing meditation you've learned a few lessons back trains us to do just that. To notice when we've strayed and redirect us to get back on track in the moment. It's an ideal preparation to notice in real life when you've strayed in your life, and gently redirect yourself in the right direction. Even the most experienced meditator will eventually stray from his breath. He'll notice it and gently redirect himself back to his goal.

Valued living is very similar to this meditation. No matter how dedicated, you'll eventually find yourself straying off your values. The trick, the true achievement, is in noticing when you've strayed from your values and redirecting yourself back to them. You pause and you notice the disconnection from your values and make a gentle return. You do this as many times as it takes. Persistent return to a valued pattern of living is the true heart of commitment. Commitment lives and breathes in the moment of return.

Remember these three rules.

Success is determined by whether you kept the assigned task, not whether it was easy or hard, comfortable or uncomfortable, or urge-free or urge-filled.

During the exercise, you should be open to experiencing all urges, feelings, thoughts, or emotions freely and fully, even if they aren't pleasant.

Remember that the point of this exercise is not to make you feel better. It is to challenge you to commit to a course of behavior and make room in your mind for whatever shows up.

ZORG THE ALIEN

I'd like you to meet Zorg. He's an alien from a faraway galaxy who's traveling the universe to learn about other life-forms. In his travels, Zorg has met humans, and he knows that these amazing creatures have these things called values that guide the way they go through life. On this visit, Zorg has chosen you as his subject of study. He's up in space in his ship with a huge telescope focused on you, and he's just observing what you do.

Let's suppose that Zorg has seen your list of values and valued actions. He knows what you value and how you'd behave if you were living according to those values.

For the purposes of his study, and relying solely on observation of your behavior, Zorg has to score how much he thinks you're living according to your values. Remember, he can only see how you act, not how you wish to act.

Based on that, how do you think Zorg would score you in the life domains we've discussed? Let's say his scale goes from 0 to 10, with 0 meaning you aren't acting at all according to your values and 10 meaning that your actions are fully consistent with your values. What score do you think Zorg would give you? Now think about the scores you'd like Zorg to give you. Let's go through all the domains again so you can say how you'd like to score in each.

How Commitment Directly Relates To Your Porn Addiction

As a member of the NoPorn Plan you've commitment yourself to stay off porn and do productive things instead. There are three questions that will help you commit to your values:

- Where will the commitment take place?
- What you are committing to doing?
- What tools can you use to help you keep this commitment?

Instructions: Please list and describe as many situations as you can think of when your urges to watch porn or porn-filled thoughts are likely to occur.

Also consider situations in which porn use or trying to control your urges directly affected your ability to carry out valued behaviors. What valued activity could you commit to doing, regardless if your urges show up?

Committed action is choosing to stand in the presence of distressing or unwanted thoughts, feelings, memories, or sensations that arise while engaging in actions that embody personal values. For example, when you feel the urge to do porn, you just will use a technique we'll teach you in the next lesson called Urge Surfing and engage in committed action by choosing to do something else instead.

FINALLY, ASK YOURSELF THESE QUESTIONS:

Am I willing to make room for the difficult thoughts and feelings that show up without getting caught up in them or struggling with them?

Am I willing to take effective action in order to do what, deep in my heart, matters?

If your answer is yes, go ahead and give it a go. If your answer is no, consider these three questions:

- Does this really and truly matter to you? 1.
- If it does, then what is the cost to you of avoiding it or putting it off?
- Would you rather have the life-draining pain of staying stuck or the life-enhancing pain of moving forward?

[13]

Master Your Time And Structure Your Life To Kick Porn Out Of It

IT HAS BEEN FOUND that unstructured time is the number one cause of porn-relapses (Maltz & Maltz, 2010). When I was addicted to porn, whenever I had nothing better to do my mind would automatically go to porn because at that point it was the easiest thing for my mind to access.

Minds are almost never still (Unless you're in very deep meditation) and they have to be occupied with something, and as such if you don't have anything specific to do your mind will turn to pornography.

That's why in the **MAGIC** Process you've created a list of tasks to keep you occupied forever. Now we'll simply organize them in such a way that you'll know to do in every moment of your life, so that there simply won't be any place for porn in your life, period.

THE EXECUTIVE VS THE WORKER

Now to get a bit academic here I will tell you something about working memory. When you try to plan out things at the same time as when you do them you're working at 50% of your capacity. This is because your working memory (The RAM of your brain for those computer geeks out there) is very limited and when half of it taken up trying to come up with what to do and the other half is occupied by porn it's impossible to be productive. That's why it's important for you to plan out your day, week and month before it starts.

You're already on your way to do just that since after you completed the **MAGIC** process you ended up with a list of specific tasks. Right now you just have to make them even more specific so that you can make them into very tangible to do's. You do that by chunking. Let's say I have a task such as; "I need write an essay for school". This could be broken down into several smaller and more manageable tasks such as:

- **Note out research for your paper**
- **Write an outline for your paper**
- **Write the paper**
- **Proofread your essay**

The number one rule of task creation is to make them as specific and 'chunked down' as possible.

Now let's discuss the second rule of task creation. That is to Always include a **VERB** in your to do's.

Let's look at this task:

Email

This doesn't really tell you anything. Now let's check this task:

Check your email

This is a specific and imaginable task. Avoid 'saving time' by writing up ambiguous tasks in your to do's. Always include a verb in your to do's. This will make them tangible, imaginable, and achievable.

The third rule of structuring your life is to differentiate habits, rituals and to do's.

Rituals (So called dailies by some) are things that you do every day, every week or every month like:

- Meditating using one of the meditations from the NoPorn Plan
- Exercising
- Writing if you're a writer
- Go to church on Sunday

Habits are things that cannot be defined by time and are simply practices for behavior. Such as:

- Eating healthy
- Mindfully eating all your meals
- Writing down a dream after you wake up

To do's are things you do one time and then 'cross them over'
For example here are mine:
Proof read lesson 27 of the Noporn plan (Remember they have to be as specific as possible)
Outline the video for lesson 27
Record the meditation for lesson 27

Now you might think to yourself "Gee that's all well and good but how will implement all of this?" There's a free piece of software that will plan your life out in this way AND increase your motivation and commitment at the same time It's called Habitica.

This program will let you not only plan out all of your tasks, habits, and rituals it will also create a system of rewards. Life is not all about worth. It's okay to indulge in benign pleasurable activities such as reading or watching an occasional movie when you have done the work. By putting all your rewards in Habitica and committing to do them only when you've 'bought them' in this program you're ensuring that your pleasure is never a 'guilty pleasure' but an <u>earned pleasure</u>. To learn more simply visit https://habitica.com

Now you might be asking yourself; "How do I transfer my to do list to Habitica without making it overwhelming?"

After doing the magic process with all of your tasks you've probably ended up with a very long list of tasks. The secret that will make it far less overwhelming is to put them in a separate document and save it somewhere safe. You can download and install Dropbox and upload your document there. Dropbox has become a mandatory program in today's world, and it can become really handy. Once you're done, now create your first ritual. Put your tasks from your task list into Habitica. Now every week you'll essentially transfer your tasks from your task list into your Habitica to do list. You'll only put the tasks into Habitica that you can do this week. Not next week or the week after that, just this week. That way you won't be overwhelmed by an unnecessarily long list of tasks; remember that you must live in the present.

Whenever you spontaneously come up with an urgent task during the week simply add it to Habitica. And whenever you come up with any non-urgent tasks (For example something that has to get done but it can get done in a month or two) you'll put it into your task list document.

Now organize the tasks in Habitica's to do list in order of priority. The urgent and important tasks should be accomplished first, followed by others in order of importance and chronology. You can also group tasks together by creating 'checklists' inside of tasks. That way you'll always know what to do.

Now you might say "This is all well and good. But this really doesn't plan out my day."

This is the weak point of Habitica. But that doesn't mean one cannot remedy it. We'll do that by combining Habitica with the most powerful daily time management system ever created; <u>The Pomodoro Technique</u> (You can learn more at http://pomodorotechnique.com/).

The science behind this is simple. Humans have been proved to be able to continuously focus for only 25 minutes. After that our minds get distracted, and we might start thinking about porn. Additionally our minds can only effectively focus on one thing at a time. This is again because our working memory is limited and when it's over-encumbered your IQ decreases. It has been shown that when you multitask your IQ decreases by about 30%.

The solution to this problem is to work continuously <u>On One Task</u> and forget <u>Everything Else</u> in your life. You just work on this one thing and forget about everything else.

This is what The Pomodoro Technique is all about. You work for 25 minutes (or 10-20 minutes if your attention span is shorter due to excessive use of pornography and video games) then take a break for 2-5 minutes. Then after 4-7 work sessions you take a longer break for 30 minutes to use up the reward points in Habitica.

The great thing is that The Pomodoro Technique has many desktop apps. My favorite is Pomodone (You can learn more about it at is official website: http://pomodoneapp.com/)

Since Habitica is an online program and as such it might conflict with the power block method (As seen back in Chapter 2) The alternative is to use the Habitica mobile app on a smartphone with an internet filter. But the better alternative is to do this:

Each day before your internet gets turned down by your preffered power block method transfer the list of tasks you have to accomplish the next day into yet another desktop app. (Both Pomodairo which works everywhere allows you to create a Pomodoro to-do list). Don't make any chunk larger than 7 pomodoros. If a tasks takes longer than 7 hours to complete it means it can be chunked down.

Alternatively you can also transfer these tasks into a pomodoro application installed on your smartphone. Many pomodoro applications will have the option to create a task list. If you have a smartphone though you can use a pomodoro application without a task list and just use the task list in Habitica.

This way you'll have your entire day planned out to the letter leaving no time to porn.

The pomodoro technique will turn anything you do into a meditation in essence. The key to using this technique is:

- Have a very specific thing to do during every block of time.
- Focus only on that one thing.
- Whenever you're distracted by anything else. Notice it and move your attention right back down.

Do you remember the mindfulness of breathing meditation you listened to a while back? This is similar. It's just an 'easier' version of it since chances are what you'll be working on will be easier to attend to than your breath. Essentially any activity that you give full attention to and come back to immediately after you notice that you were distracted, counts as meditation.

Today I will give you yet another meditation to make you aware of this.

MINDFULNESS OF A CHORE

Pick any activity that you do automatically that's part of your morning routine. It could be brushing your teeth, shaving, or taking a shower. When you do it, become fully present with it and focus completely on what you're doing. Become aware of all the sensations accompanying that activity. Become aware of what you feel, what you hear and what you see while doing this activity. Become fully present with it and welcome everything you experience while doing it. For example when you're in the shower notice the temperature of the water and how it feels on your skin, and allow yourself to notice the sound the water makes. Notice the smell of the soap, and the way it feels on your skin. Notice the sight of the water droplets hitting your skin, and the water dripping down your body, notice the steam rising upwards. Become aware and feel the movements of your arms as you scrub your skin. When thoughts arise acknowledge them, notice them, and let them be, and very gently bring your attention back to the shower. Whenever you attention will inevitably wander just allow yourself to gently acknowledge it, note what distracted you, and bring your attention back to the shower. You can also do this with every possible chore such as doing the dishes or any other menial chore.

Just pick any chore you'd normally rush through and 'get over with' and aim to do this chore as a mindfulness practice. This is actually a very common practice found in Zen Monasteries. When Zen Monks do anything from cooking to chopping wood, they do it as a mindfulness practice.

For example when you wash the dishes notice the color of the dishes and the feel of the soap or dish-glove on your skin. Notice the sound the dishes make as you clean them. Notice the smell of the cleaning solution. Notice the movement of your hands on the dishes and notice the feeling of the sponge in your hand.

LAST BUT NOT LEAST – NEVER BEAT YOURSELF UP

Many porn addicts have a self-defeating all or nothing attitude towards life. They think that they need to do everything perfectly in order to be a 'success'. After going through this course for quite a bit you already know that this is not true. But it's important to internalize this.

That's why in future lessons we'll introduce you to yet another therapeutic practice. It's called self-compassion meditation and it's specifically designed to make YOU your best friend. Self-compassion is a skill that's proven to not only improve interpersonal relationships (you cannot have a proper relationship with other people unless you have one with yourself) but it has also been proven to alleviate many addictions. Whenever we release we tend to beat ourselves up which in turn strengthens our addiction. The correct attitude towards a relapse, slip or a failed goal is one of forgiveness and compassion which today's meditation will train, and will prevent you from being overwhelmed and burning yourself out with leading a productive life.

[14]

How To Conquer Your Urges With Urge Surfing

URGES TO USE PORN are very hard to control or 'eliminate' and although some eastern yogis did attempt that and largely succeeded. They did that by removing their whole libido. While I will teach you how they did that in a future lesson, right now I will teach you a simple technique that will take power away from your pornographic urges, so that you'll no longer be controlled by porn. (Bowen, Chawla, & Marlatt, 2010)

URGE SURFING

Before I describe it to you, I want you to look at the concept of urges. Whenever you feel an urge you essentially only have two choices: To act upon it, or not to act upon it. And as such whenever you have an urge you need to ask yourself: "If I act on this urge, will I be acting like the person I want to be? Will it help me take my life in the direction I want to go?" If the answer is yes, then it makes sense for you to act on that urge. For example, if you haven't eaten in two days and have the urge to eat you might eat something.

On the other hand if you have the urge to use pornography, this urge is not in alignment with who you want to be, and as such it's best not to act on it.

Whenever you're triggered your porn patterns are activated; the thoughts and beliefs that cause you to do porn have been given precedence in your mind. They are well trained, so well trained that whenever they are triggered they can take control of your entire mind if you fuse with them. At that point you run on automatic pilot, and are essentially controlled by them (Williams & MA, 2012). Whenever you're triggered by an outside stimulus a well-trained porn pattern is activated and you act on automatic pilot. Acting on automatic pilot is essentially mindlessness and fusion. You fuse with your pornified thought.

The solution to this problem is to practice mindfulness either with the technique you'll learn in this lesson called Urge Surfing or with the technique you'll learn in the a further lesson called TAP.

To Conquer Your Porn Patterns You'll Have to Notice Your Urges

To handle your urges effectively you first have to become aware of them and acknowledge them. Chances are that through the intensive mindfulness training given to you in previous lessons you've already become aware of your urges. Now you just have to learn to acknowledge the urge whenever you notice it. It's very simple to do.

You just silently say to yourself "I'm having the urge to do x"

Such as "I'm having the urge to use porn"

Then simply check your values. "Will acting on this urge help me be the person I want to be? Will it help me take my life in the direction I want?" If the answer is yes, then go ahead and act on it, use the urge to give you momentum. But if the answer is no, then instead take an action that's more in line with your values.

So what do we do when an urge pushes us into the opposite direction of our values? We don't want to struggle or resist that urge, because that just makes it stronger and makes it impossible for us to take effective action. So rather than trying to resist or suppress it one has to open up to it. By opening up to it and making room for it you'll take the power of the urge away. It will no longer control you, as you'll have the space needed to make correct choices about your life.

To help you do that we've integrated everything you've learned so far about mindfulness and values into one simple technique called urge surfing, which you'll use from now on every time an urge to use porn arises.

Have you ever watched ocean waves? A wave starts off small and gently grows. Then it slowly gathers speed and increases in size. Then it continues to expand and until it reaches its maximum size. Then once it has reached its peak size, it gradually becomes smaller. The same happens with urges in your body. They start of small and then gradually increase in size.

If you give an ocean wave enough space, it will reach its peak size and harmlessly subside. But what happens when a wave encounters resistance? Have you ever seen a wave crash onto a beach or smash against rocks? It's loud, and destructive.

In urge surfing, you learn not to resist the urge waves that happen in your mind. Instead you'll simply surf on them until they dissipate on their own or until they'll lose all control over you.

I have further improved upon urge surfing by integrating it with the NoPorn phrase. That's why I call my technique Urge Surfing +.

Let's now guide you through urge surfing + step by step:

1.   First you watch. Just notice what you feel in your body.

2.   Then you acknowledge the feeling you're having for example "I'm having the urge to use porn"

3.   Notice your breathing and ask yourself "Could I open up to this experience?" Allow yourself to simply make room for this experience.

4.   Rate it. For example: "I have the urge to use porn, and it's now a 7" This will allow you to defuse from it a bit.

5.   Then ask yourself: "Could I allow this experience to be as it in this moment?" "Could I allow myself to observe it like a curious scientist?" Just observe it. Remember that no matter how huge that wave gets, you have room for it. If you give it enough space its power over you will subside. Just observe it, and open up to it. Create space for it.

6.   I want you to re-align yourself with your values by saying the NoPorn phrase out loud or silently to yourself "I choose to be porn free"

Then you'll consult your values. Just ask yourself "What action can I make right now instead of trying to resist or control my urges- that will enhance my life in the long term?"

Then you just TAKE ACTION. On that thing from point 6

In other words, to manage your urges effectively, you need to ACT:

•   A = Accept your thoughts and feelings.
•   C = Connect with your values.
•   T = Take effective action.

Urge surfing is a skill, and like any skill it requires practice. You'll now expected to practice urge surfing whenever an urge to use porn arises, and from now on your daily inventory will prompt you to describe your experience with this technique. It also would be a great idea to practice urge surfing with any other urge that comes up: the urge to use chocolate, the urge to overeat. Anything. By practicing urge surfing on unrelated urges you'll increase your proficiency with it enough to tackle even your strongest pornographic urges.

In a later lesson we'll integrate this urge surfing technique with other techniques you'll learn in this course to create an even-more powerful technique just in case your pornographic urges are so powerful that urge surfing doesn't seem to be enough. But for now I want you to use urge surfing on it's own whenever you have an urge to do anything: An urge for chocolate, sweets, TV, video games and of course porn etc. Practicing it in such a way will train you to use it whenever you have an urge. This will make sure that you'll remember to use it when you have an urge to watch porn or masturbate.

EXERCISE: URGE SURFING

You can get a recorded version in my course. Since you're so far into this book I want to reward you with a 75% off coupon which you can get it by submitting your email to http://nopornplan.com

First you watch. Just notice what you feel in your body.

Then you acknowledge the feeling you're having for example: "I'm having the urge to use porn"

Now put your attention on your breath and yourself "Could I open up to this experience?" Allow yourself to simply make room for this experience. Just see if you could make room for it.

Pause For 5 Seconds

Now rate it. How strong is it on a scale from 1-10. You can rate it silently or out loud.

Now ask yourself "Could I allow this experience to be as it in this moment?" And see what happens are you able to be with this experience. To just observe it nonjudgmentally?

Pause For 5 Seconds

Now ask yourself:

"Could I allow myself to observe it like a curious scientist?" And just observe it. Remember that no matter how huge those urges get, you have room for it. If you give it enough space its power over you will subside. Just observe it, and open up to it. Create space for it.

Pause For 10 Seconds

I will give you a few seconds to just be with this urge.

Pause For 10 Seconds

Now we would like you to consult your values. Just ask yourself "What action can I make right now instead of trying to resist or control my urges- that will enhance my life in the long term?" And now just do that thing!

[15]

Tap Out The Porn With The Porn Tap

TAP is our flagship relapse prevention technique that builds upon everything you've learned so far about:

- **Mindfulness**
- **Acupressure Desensitization**
- **And relapse prevention**

In a sense it's a more advanced version of the Urge surfing technique you've learned in the previous lesson.

THE PORN TAP STEP BY STEP

Let's discuss the step of **TAAP** in greater detail. The First Step is to simply **TAP**.

When you have the urge to do porn your automatic response should be to stimulate your acupressure points. This will break the pattern currently in motion and allow you to clear your mind sufficiently to respond in a present and mindful way.

You have practiced acupressure desensitization previously and by this point you should be familiar with it enough so that stimulating your acupoints can become something you do automatically each time you feel a porn urge coming up.

You can stimulate your acupoints either using the full **AD** sequence or **PAD**. We recommend **PAD** since it's shorter and you can use it in public without looking weird.

The Second Step is to accept what is and become mindful.

1.   Observe the sensations that are happening in your body and any emotions, moods or thoughts you are having. Just notice as much as you can about your experience with willingness and acceptance

2.   Focus on your breathing. Use it as an anchor.

3.   Then expand your awareness to include the rest of your body, your experience and see if you can gently hold it in your awareness

This step of **TAP** is essentially Urge Surfing. Nothing more nothing less. The point is for you to become present with your urges instead of reacting to them on automatic pilot. The Last Step Is to realign your mind into Productivity. This part is itself composed of 3 steps:

- Affirm
- Ask
- Alternative

Let's explain each one step by step

Affirm

If you're working on your porn addiction you can use your NoPorn Phrase: "I choose to be porn free". If you want to use **TAP** for more than porn addiction you can use the phrase you learned in the self-esteem exercise: "I choose to be the best me I can be"

Ask

You can ask yourself these questions to make this process easier:
- Is doing what my mind tells me to do in alignment with my values? (For example: Is using porn in alignment with my values?)
- Will doing this help me live a more valued life?
- Will doing this improve my life in the long term?

The Last Step Is a Productive Alternative

Simply ask yourself: What's a productive alternative that's aligned with my values that I can do right now instead of doing what my mind tells me to do?

(In your case: What's a productive alternative that's aligned with my values that I can do right now instead watching porn?)

And then simply do that thing instead.

This technique is simple and will put your mind back on track to living a value-filled life.

So Here's the NoPorn Tap in a Nutshell:
- TAP
- Accept
- Productive alternative (Composed of 3 As 1: Affirm. 2: Ask. 3: Productive Alternative)

LEARN ABOUT YOUR PORN PATTERNS TO PREVENT RELAPSES FOREVER

When an average Joe is triggered by an outside stimulus he acts on autopilot because he's unable to defuse from his automatic thoughts and feelings.

This is especially evident in porn addiction. In the NoPorn Plan we call the automatic program that is responsible for your porn addiction the <u>Porn Pattern</u>. Let's look at how it works.

An average Joe sees a sexy billboard or sees something sexy on facebook and the porn pattern in his brain gets immediately activated, it conjures beliefs and thoughts and an average person fuses with them and relapses, which in turn creates judgmental thoughts such as "Oh no... I've been so bad" the guilt caused by fusion with these thought fuels yet another relapse

But you're not an average Joe now. You have learned tools that 99% of people don't even know or has heard about. You're no longer average. You're above average. Because of that a new possibility is given to you.

When you're triggered instead of fusing with the thoughts and beliefs conjured by your old activated mind programs you can use **TAP** to defuse from them and respond with awareness. This is beautifully illustrated in the following diagram:

Porn Pattern Picture

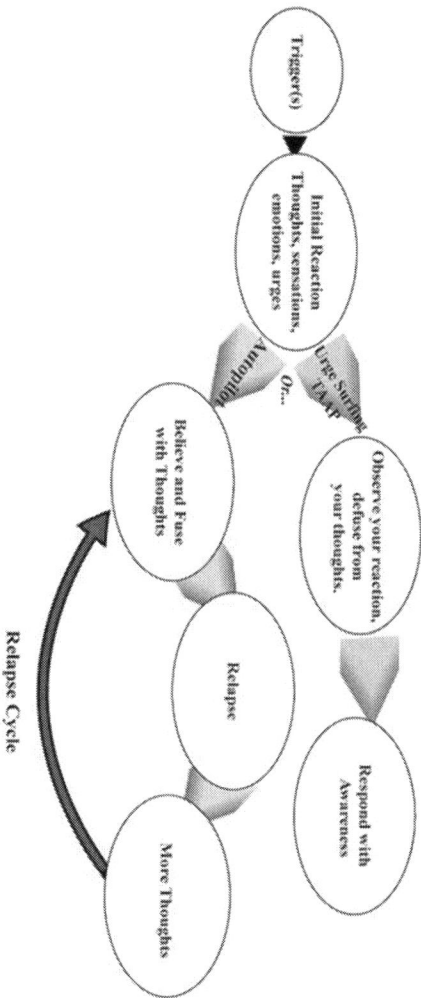

Triggers(s)

Initial Reaction
Thoughts, sensations,
emotions, urges

Autopilot

Or...

Urge Surfing
TAMP

Believe and Fuse
with Thoughts

Observe your reaction,
defuse from
your thoughts.

Relapse

Respond with
Awareness

More Thoughts

Relapse Cycle

It's important for you to understand your porn patterns and plan out your reaction to them. Here's my porn pattern

Matt's Porn Pattern Picture

Print out this worksheet and think of a situation that had trigger(s) and/or led to a porn relapse in the past. Write out the trigger(s), your initial reaction that followed, and the events in the ovals below.

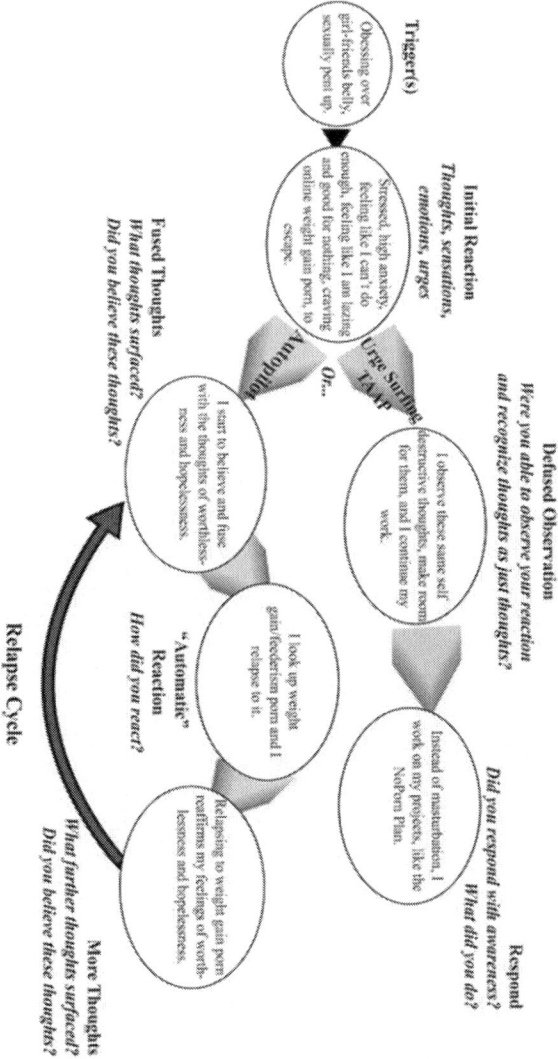

Trigger(s)
Obsessing over girl-friends belly, sexually pent up.

Initial Reaction
Thoughts, sensations, emotions, urges
Stressed, high anxiety, feeling like I can't do enough, feeling like I am lazing and good for nothing, craving online weight gain porn, to escape.

Fused Thoughts
What thoughts surfaced? Did you believe these thoughts?
I start to believe and fuse with the thoughts of worthlessness and hopelessness.

Absorption

Urge Surfing
Or...
I AM

Defused Observation
Were you able to observe your reaction and recognize thoughts as just thoughts?
I observe these same self destructive thoughts, make room for them, and I continue my work.

Respond
Did you respond with awareness? What did you do?
Instead of masturbation, I work on my projects, like the NoFom Plan.

"Automatic" Reaction
How did you react?
I look up weight gain feederism porn and I relapse to it.

More Thoughts
What further thoughts surfaced? Did you believe these thoughts?
Relapsing to weight gain porn reaffirms my feelings of worthlessness and hopelessness.

Relapse Cycle

Now in todays' exercise you'll be asked to print out and fill out a diagram in which you'll fill out your own porn pattern. Simply print it or edit it using your favorite photo editing program.

Your Porn Pattern Picture

Print out this worksheet and think of a situation that had triggered(s) and/or led to a porn relapse in the past. Write out the trigger(s), your initial reaction that followed, and the events in the ovals below.

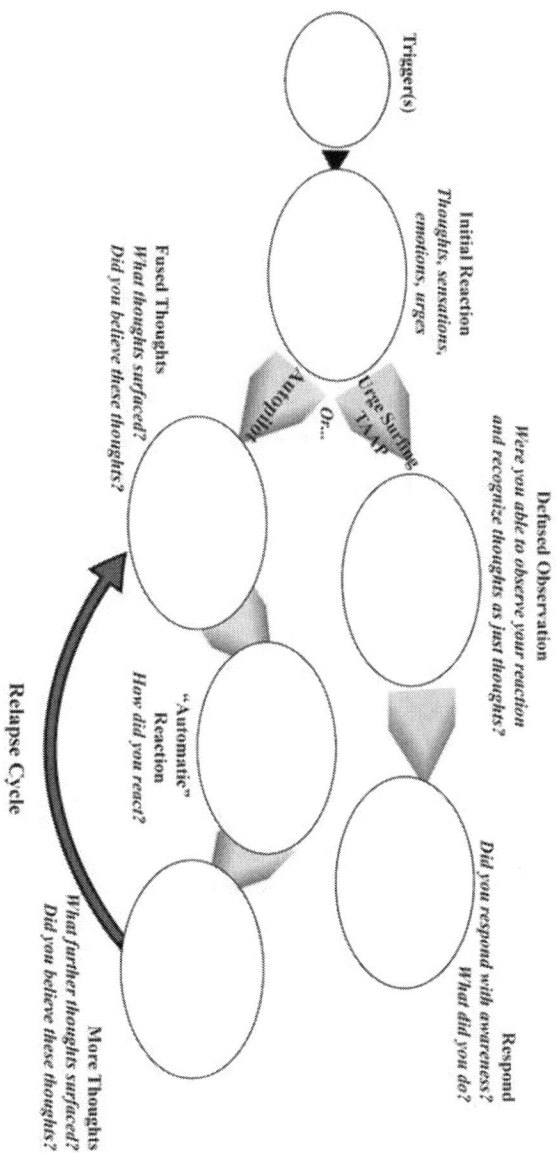

Trigger(s)

Initial Reaction
Thoughts, sensations, emotions, urges

Acceptance Or... **Urge Surfing TAAP**

Defused Observation
Were you able to observe your reaction and recognize thoughts as just thoughts?

Fused Thoughts
What thoughts surfaced? Did you believe these thoughts?

"Automatic" Reaction
How did you react?

Respond
Did you respond with awareness? What did you do?

Relapse Cycle

More Thoughts
What further thoughts surfaced? Did you believe these thoughts?

Fill out the lower part of the worksheet your own experiences with relapses. Fill out the upper part of the worksheet with how you'll react once you'll consistently apply tap for your cravings.

What thoughts and beliefs are conjured each time you're triggered by porn?

What's the automatic reaction to them?

After you relapse, what further thoughts surface? Do you believe these thoughts?

What would happen if instead of reacting to them to your triggers on autopilot you'd reacted to them with mindfulness by using **TAAAP.**

What would happen if, thanks to **TAAAP**, you were able to observe your reaction and recognize thoughts as just thoughts?

Would you be able to respond with awareness? What would you do?

There's yet another aspect of relapse prevention that you need to master. As you saw in the diagram our relapses are fueled by us beating ourselves up for our relapses. Being ashamed and feeling guilty about what we've done increases our stress levels which in turn makes us more likely to relapse in the future.

To counteract this you'll need to learn yet another skill. It's called self-compassion.

Self-compassion is different from self-esteem. Self-compassion is an attitude of being your own best friend, developing this attitude will not only improve your mindfulness practice but also your productivity, your emotional stability and your ability to relate to others. Because you really can't be compassionate to other people until you learn to be compassionate to yourself.

[16]

How To Move From Pornified Sexuality To Authentic Intimacy

MANY PORN ADDICTS FEEL AFRAID about returning to sexual activity. This is understandable. For some porn addicts, sex acts as a porn trigger and makes them relapse, while for others sex and porn are separate and they are able to have sex while still being free from porn.

In order to be able to be sexually active while remaining porn free, you need to clearly differentiate between porn and sex. To do this, you need to develop a completely new intimacy–oriented approach to sex (Maltz & Maltz, 2010).

An intimacy-oriented approach to sex allows you to experience dimensions of sexuality that porn doesn't allow you to experience. In this lesson, you'll learn a number of exercises and practices that will help you make the transition from pornified sexuality to intimacy based sexuality.

PORN DOESN'T PREPARE YOU FOR SEX

At the end of the day porn is all about fantasy. A real life sexual encounter is completely different from what one experiences while masturbating to pixels on a screen. Many porn users think that because they have to avoid porn they have to avoid all forms of sexuality. This is not true. Our goal in this part of your recovery is to learn how to express your sexuality without the use of pornography.

UNDERSTAND THE DIFFERENCE BETWEEN PORN AND SEX

Porn teaches us that sex is very mechanical and competitive. To overcome porn, you have to approach sex as an intimacy practice. You do that by realizing the difference between pornified sexuality and intimate sexuality. You'll also achieve that through the use of mindfulness skills.

When you allow yourself to fully get into the experience of sex, getting back into it each time you're distracted by pornographic thoughts, you'll learn to experience true healthy sexuality.

Pornified sex	Intimate sexuality
• Sex is using someone	o Sex is always respectful
• Sex is "doing to" someone	o Sex has ethical boundaries
• Sex is a performance for others	o Sex requires morals and values
• Sex is compulsive	o Sex requires honesty
• Sex is a public commodity	o Sex involves all the senses
• Sex requires a double life	o Sex is lasting satisfaction
• Sex is separate from love	o Sex is caring for someone
• Sex is watching others	o Sex is sharing with a partner
• Sex can be hurtful	o Sex is nurturing
• Sex is emotionally distant	o Sex requires certain conditions
• Sex can happen anytime	o Sex is safe
• Sex is unsafe	o Sex enhances self-esteem
• Sex can be degrading	o Sex is a private experience
• Sex can be irresponsible	o Sex is an expression of love
• Sex is based on visual imagery	o Sex is approached responsibly
• Sex is devoid of morality	o Sex enhances who you really are
• Sex involves deception	o Sex is emotionally close
• Sex lacks healthy communication	o Sex requires healthy communication
• Sex has no ethical limits	o Sex is a natural drive
• Sex compromises your values	o Sex is about genuine connection
• Sex feels shameful	o Sex is a personal treasure
• Sex is impulse gratification	o Sex reflects your values

PAVE THE WAY FOR INTIMACY

It's always a good idea to pave the way for intimacy during sex. Simply become physically attuned to your partner by massaging his/her back or doing other sensual activities.

If you have a partner learn to talk about sex. You have to learn to talk about sex in an honest way. In porn, no one says that they are uncomfortable with something. Nor do they have any other kind of healthy sexual dialogue. It's also important to be honest about sex and to talk about sex with your partner being able to honestly talk about sex is important to your sexual health. But at the same it's important to remember that becoming comfortable with talking about sex takes effort and practice.

You'll also have to realize that you'll need to let go of certain unrealistic expectations created by porn that might be damaging to your partner ant to your relationship. You do this by discussing sex with your partner using the topics outlined below.

TOPICS FOR CREATING INTIMATE SEX

- What do you enjoy most about sex?
- What feelings do you hope to experience when you are sexual?
- What do you identify as the purpose and meaning of sex in your life?
- How do you feel about yourself as a sexual person?
- How has porn influenced your sexuality?
- What past experiences may be affecting how you feel about sex now? For example: Have you ever had a sexually transmitted disease? Have you been troubled by chronic sexual functioning problems? Do you have a past history of sexual abuse?

- What are your preferences for when, where, and how you would most like to engage in sex?
- How do you like your partner to initiate sex?
- What things get you in the mood? How do you show that you are interested in having sex?
- What type of language do you prefer when discussing body parts and sexual activities? For example, are you comfortable with slang terms or do you prefer medical terminology, or something in between?
- How do you want to protect against unwanted pregnancy and sexually transmitted infections?
- What do you need to feel physically safe and comfortable when you relate sexually? For example: cleanliness, nail care, privacy, pillows, or lubricants.
- What do you like to do following a sexual experience in order to continue feeling positive and intimate?
- What are your expectations regarding confidentiality, fidelity, and the future of your sexual relationship?

You may want to consider the following set of guidelines that many couples in recovery decide to honor:
- It's okay to ask for what we each want.
- Ridicule, even disguised as teasing, is not allowed.
- It's okay for either of us to say "no" to a particular kind of touch or sex at any time.
- It's okay to stop and take breaks in our sexual interaction at any time.
- Our needs for comfort and safety are a priority and will be addressed as needed.
- We equally value emotional closeness and physical pleasure.
- Expand your sensory awareness to increase your intimacy

Porn is 100% visual. And it has the potential to desensitize us from the physical experience of sex. It makes us less present during sex, which in turn makes us ejaculate more quickly and makes us unable to both give and receive pleasure from our partner.

The way to rectify this is the practice mindfulness in bed. Whenever you have sex, treat it as mindfulness practice. Allow you to be fully present in the experience, and whenever a pornographic thought comes up, gently re-align yourself to the sexual act. All the other mindfulness exercises in this course prepare you for this.

YOU'LL HAVE TO LEARN TO LOOK LOVINGLY AT YOUR PARTNER

Past porn use has trained you to look at a person like an object. This causes your partner to retreat and makes all the people you stare at uneasy.

Ask yourself: Are you looking at your partner the same way you looked at porn images, or are you looking at him/her in a way that conveys caring and respect?

Remember: Unlike a porn picture, a partner has a reaction to the way you look at him/her.

Try asking your partner how they feel when you look at them in different situations.

[17]

Learn How To Transform Sexual Energy Into Productivity With The NoPorn Diet

In this last lesson you'll get a crash course in the sexual sublimation process of the yogis. Ancient yogis were forced to be celibate and as such they had to create processes to curb their libido. The body was seen as secret in those cultures and as such castration wasn't an option. Instead they used yoga, pranayama and diet to turn their sexual drive into a spiritual drive. Similarly you can use sexual transmutation to turn sexuality into productivity

The processes are composed of three steps:

1: Having a clear purpose in life: Which is essentially knowing your values and fully living by them.

2: Practicing a diet that lowers your libido: We have our own proprietary blend of this called the NoPorn diet, which we'll describe in this lesson.

3: Practicing regular physical exercise: Although yoga is preferred as it is specifically designed to assist you with that, especially the sivananda school of yoga.

HAVING A CLEAR PURPOSE IN LIFE

We we've had a whole module about values and commitment. And as such you should have a clear idea now what your life is all about. But we can clarify that again. "What's your life purpose? What's the one thing that's more important to your life than anything else?" What's your drive? Whenever you want to watch porn, just do what you value instead.

PRACTICE THE NOPORN DIET

This is a proprietary technique that took me years to develop. It's based on a diet given to yogis, Taoist monks, and other spiritual seekers, in order for them to become celibate. (Cousens, 2009)
The old ancient traditions explained the efficiency of that practice in terms of 'energies' and other fluff stuff. But in reality that practice is very simple.(Sivananda,1960)/ It's simply a low-fat diet composed primarily of whole grains, fruits and veggies.(Graham, 2006). The truth is that for you to have normal testosterone levels you need to get at least 25% of your calories from fat. When you lower that number to 10% or 9% your libido drops, because your testosterone levels drop. It's that simple. So essentially:
Eat less than 10% of your calories from fat while having an at least a 25% calorie deficiency and your libido will drop.

Here's the summary of this diet. You essentially:
- Eat 30-60% of your calories from vegetables
- 10-40% calories from fruit
- About 20% calories from potatoes and whole grains
- 0-10% calories from nuts, seeds and avocados
- 0-10% calories from beans and legumes. (These contain fats. You can eat unlimited amounts of dried soy

cutlets which are dehydrated and have fat removed from them).

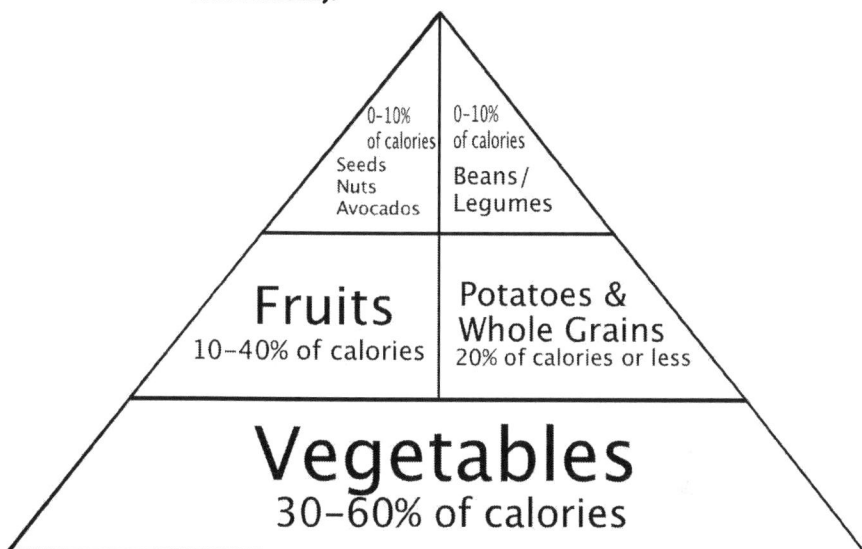

0-10% of calories
Seeds
Nuts
Avocados

0-10% of calories
Beans/
Legumes

Fruits
10–40% of calories

Potatoes &
Whole Grains
20% of calories or less

Vegetables
30–60% of calories

This is of course not the only diet that would work. Any diet that has less than 10% calories from fat while sustaining a caloric deficit will work for the purposes of lowering your libido. One has to note that this diet is very hard to practice in real life without the support of one of the programs I recommended to you above, and as such you should only use it if you feel that you

WHERE TO GO FROM HERE

Congratulations! You've finished this book. All you need to do now is to practice it.

I suggest that you subscribe to my blog at http://nopornplan.com. In it I post comics about recovering from porn addiction which will help you further.

Additionally I'm currently working on books about increasing your sexual stamina and how to master dating and relationships. If you're interested in those please go to http://nopornplan.com and signup to our email list. You will get the books for free when they launch.

Where you'll be able to sign up on the early bird list and receive the ebook versions of those books for free when they launch

Additionally since you've finished this book I'll give you 75% of my udemy course which is a companion to this book. You just have to sign up at http://nopornplan.com and you will get the 75% off coupon right away.

Bibliography

-Alquist, J. L., & Baumeister, R. F. (2012). Self-control and addiction. In H. J. Shaffer, D. A. LaPlante, & S. E. Nelson (Eds.), APA addiction syndrome handbook, Vol. 1: Foundations, influences, and expressions of addiction. (pp. 165–174). Washington: American Psychological Association. Retrieved from: http://content.apa.org/books/13751-008

-Bowen, S., Chawla, N., & Marlatt, G. A. (2010). *Mindfulness-Based Relapse Prevention for Addictive Behaviors: A Clinician's Guide* (1 edition). New York: The Guilford Press.

-Byrne, R. (2006). *The secret.* New York; Hillsboro, Or.: Atria Books ; Beyond Words Pub.

-Clarkson, J., & Kopaczewski, S. (2013). Pornography Addiction and the Medicalization of Free Speech.Journal of Communication Inquiry, 37(2),128–148. http://doi.org/10.1177/0196859913482330

-Craig, G. (2011). *The EFT manual.* Santa Rosa, CA: Energy Psychology Press.

-Edelstein, M. (2009). *Three Minute Therapy.* Glenbridge Publishing Ltd.

-Ellis, A., & Ellis, D. J. (2011). *Rational Emotive Behavior Therapy* (3 edition). Washington, DC: Amer Psychological Assn.

-Feinstein, D. (2008). Energy psychology: A review of the preliminary evidence. *Psychotherapy:Theory, Research, Practice, Training,* 45(2), 199–213. http://doi.org/10.1037/0033-3204.45.2.199

-González-Menéndez, A., Fernández, P., Rodríguez, F., & Villagrá, P. (2014). Long-term outcomes of Acceptance and Commitment Therapy in drug-dependent female inmates: A randomized controlled trial. International Journal of Clinical and Health Psychology, 14(1), 18–27. http://doi.org/10.1016/S1697-2600(14)70033-X

-Harris, R. (2009). *ACT Made Simple: An Easy-To-Read Primer on Acceptance and Commitment Therapy* (1 edition). Oakland, CA: New Harbinger Publications.

-Hayes, S. C., & Smith, S. X. (2005). *Get out of your mind & into your life: the new acceptance & commitment therapy.* Oakland, CA: New Harbinger Publications.

-Kabat-Zinn, J. (2012). *Mindfulness for beginners: reclaiming the present moment--and your life.* Boulder, CO: Sounds True.

-Kelly, M. M., Sido, H., Forsyth, J. P., Ziedonis, D. M., Kalman, D., & Cooney, J. L. (2015). Acceptance and Commitment Therapy Smoking Cessation Treatment for Veterans with Posttraumatic Stress Disorder: A Pilot Study. Journal of Dual Diagnosis, 11(1), 50–55. http://doi.org/10.1080/15504263.2014.992201

-Maltz, W., & Maltz, L. (2010). *The Porn Trap: The Essential Guide to Overcoming Problems Caused by Pornography* (1 Reprint edition). New York; Enfield: William Morrow Paperbacks.

-Manson, M. (2011). *Models: Attract Women Through Honesty.* U.S.: CreateSpace Independent Publishing Platform.

-Margolis, R. D., & Zweben, J. E. (2011). Treating patients with alcohol and other drug problems: An integrated approach (2nd ed.). Washington: American Psychological Association. Retrieved from: http://content.apa.org/books/12312-000

-Mountrose, P., Mountrose, J., & Holistic Communications. (2005). *The heart & soul of EFT and beyond--: a soulful exploration of the emotional freedom techniques and holistic healing.* Arroyo Grande, Calif.: Holistic Communications.

-Owens, E. W., Behun, R. J., Manning, J. C., & Reid, R. C. (2012). The Impact of Internet Pornography on Adolescents: A Review of the Research. Sexual Addiction & Compulsivity, 19(1-2), 99–122. http://doi.org/10.1080/10720162.2012.660431

-Reich, W. (1973). *The function of the orgasm: sex-economic problems of biological energy.* New York: Noonday Press.

-Rosenberg, H., & Kraus, S. (2014). The relationship of "passionate attachment" for pornography with sexual compulsivity, frequency of use, and craving for pornography. Addictive Behaviors, 39(5), 1012–1017. http://doi.org/10.1016/j.addbeh.2014.02.010

-Sivananda, S. S. (1960). *Practice of Brahmacharya. 7th Edition: 1960.* The Yoga-Vedanta Forest Academy.

-Lowen, A. (1994). *Bioenergetics.* New York: Penguin/Arkana.

-Reich, W. (1973). *The function of the orgasm: sex-economic problems of biological energy.* New York: Noonday Press.

-Webb, C. A., Beard, C., Kertz, S. J., Hsu, K. J., & Björgvinsson, T. (2016). Differential role of CBT skills, DBT skills and psychological flexibility in predicting depressive versus anxiety symptom improvement. *Behaviour Research and Therapy, 81,* 12–20. http://doi.org/10.1016/j.brat.2016.03.006

-Watts, C., & Hilton, D. (2011). Pornography addiction: A neuroscience perspective. Surgical Neurology International, 2(1), 19. http://doi.org/10.4103/2152-7806.76977

-McDougal, B. (n.d.). Porned Out: erectile dysfunction, depression, and 7 more (selfish) reasons to quit porn. (M. Kennedy, Ed.).

-Wenrich, W., Dawley, H., & General, D. (1976). *Self-directed systematic desensitization: A guide for the student, client and therapist.* Kalamazoo, Mich: Behaviordelia.

-Williams, R. E., & MA, J. S. K. (2012). *The Mindfulness Workbook for Addiction: A Guide to Coping with the Grief, Stress and Anger that Trigger Addictive Behaviors* (Csm Wkb edition). Oakland, CA: New Harbinger Publications.

-Willis, J. (2010). *Reichian Therapy: The Technique, for Home Use.* createspace.

-Wilson, K., & DuFrene, T. (2012). *The Wisdom to Know the Difference: An Acceptance and Commitment Therapy Workbook for Overcoming Substance Abuse* (1 edition). Oakland, CA: New Harbinger Publications.

ABOUT THE AUTHOR

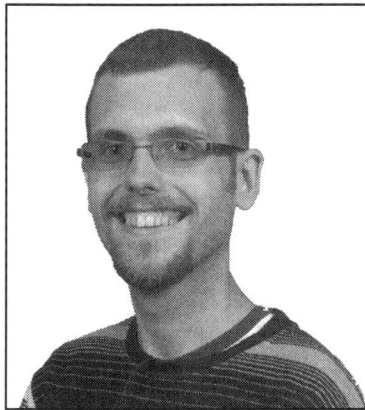

Matt Struggled with porn addiction ever since he was 12 years old. Watching it up to 6 hours per day. At age 13, he experienced his first panic attack and from that point on he tried every self-help technique and book available. But nothing helped. It only made his mental issues (including his porn addi ction) worse. Eventually rendering him catatonic for over a year. After he recovered from catatonia, Matt begun studying psychology. After graduating he became a psychologist to devote his life to giving practical, evidence-based self -help advice to people who are experiencing similar issues he had.

34288993R00148

Made in the USA
Middletown, DE
24 January 2019